Set Me Adrift
in the Sea of Faith

Rick + Cheryl
Blessings to you
and your loved
ones. Judy

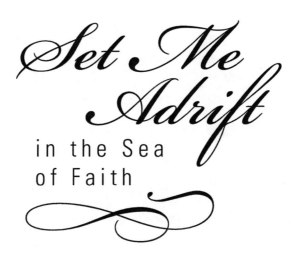

Set Me Adrift
in the Sea of Faith

The faith renewing
story of an Alzheimer
patient's daughter

Judith Ames David

TATE PUBLISHING & *Enterprises*

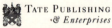

TATE PUBLISHING
 & Enterprises

Tate Publishing is committed to excellence in the publishing industry. Our staff of highly trained professionals, including editors, graphic designers, and marketing personnel, work together to produce the very finest books available. The company reflects the philosophy established by the founders, based on Psalms 68:11,

"THE LORD GAVE THE WORD AND GREAT WAS THE COMPANY OF THOSE WHO PUBLISHED IT."

If you would like further information, please contact us:
1.888.361.9473 | www.tatepublishing.com
TATE PUBLISHING & *Enterprises*, LLC | 127 E. Trade Center Terrace
Mustang, Oklahoma 73064 USA

Set Me Adrift in the Sea of Faith
Copyright © 2007 by Judith Ames David. All rights reserved.
This title is also available as a Tate Out Loud product.
Visit www.tatepublishing.com for more information

No part of this publication may be reproduced, stored in a retrieval system or transmitted in any way by any means, electronic, mechanical, photocopy, recording or otherwise without the prior permission of the author except as provided by USA copyright law.

Scripture quotations are taken from the *Holy Bible, New International Version* ®, Copyright © 1973, 1978, 1984 by International Bible Society. Used by permission of Zondervan Publishing House. All rights reserved.

This book is designed to provide accurate and authoritative information with regard to the subject matter covered. This information is given with the understanding that neither the author nor Tate Publishing, LLC is engaged in rendering legal, professional advice. Since the details of your situation are fact dependent, you should additionally seek the services of a competent professional.

Book design copyright © 2007 by Tate Publishing, LLC. All rights reserved.
Cover photo by Paul A. Preston
Cover design by Kristen Polson
Interior design by Sarah Leis

Published in the United States of America
ISBN: 978-1-5988693-9-2
07.02.09

Dedicated to the memory of Maureen Reagan for her tireless work in promoting awareness of Alzheimer's disease and giving hope for the future to its victims and their loved ones.

Acknowledgements

Special thanks to my husband Arley who patiently understands my need to write, to my brother Jon Kjellander for his analytical and computer skills, and to Joan Isom, my mentor and friend, without whose help and encouragement this book would not be possible.

Table of Contents

Foreword 11
The Dance 13
Seeds of Faith 18
Signs of Decline 25
Awakened 30
A Moving Experience 36
The Fragment of a Shell 43
A Time of Loss 48
Tears, Prayers, and Learning to Cope 55
God's Loving Gifts 61
A Place of Refuge and Hope 68
Special Moments 71
Nursing Home Angels 75
A Bit of Humor 80
Lines from the All School Play 85
Wrestling with Guilt 88
Spiritual Growth 95
A Season to Remember 100
Letting Go 104
Saying Goodbye 111
Remembering Margaret 117
A New Beginning 120
Set Me Adrift 125

Foreword
a great expression of love

As I read of a mother lying and dying with the dreadful disease Alzheimer's, I witnessed the journey of a loving daughter forced to watch helplessly as her mother wasted away with the disease that is a killer. It is no respecter of persons. Millions of people in all walks of life have Alzheimer's and/or other related dementia. Judith was able to grow in faith and wisdom as she lived with this disease that was to take her mother's life.

Although this real life story is about a very serious and devastating illness, it is tempered with love and a great deal of humor as Judith looks back on her life and a mother/daughter relationship that can't be broken by time, illness, or even death. This book should be a help and inspiration to anyone dealing with a loved one who is afflicted with Alzheimer's disease or is struggling with any life-changing event over which they have no control. Most importantly, it shows how the love of Christ can change hearts and transform lives.

> Evelyn J. Hottinger
> Medicalodge of Neosho, Missouri
> Administrator from 1994 to 2001

The Dance

Between Christmas and New Year is always a special time. It's a time to review the past year—to review your life. For me, December 2000 was even more so. The radio in my '95 Honda Accord played the usual countdown of hits from the past. Tears streamed down my face as Garth Brooks sang one of my all-time favorite songs, *The Dance*:

> And now I'm glad I didn't know
> The way it all would end the way it all would go[1]

Bittersweet memories of my mother Margaret flooded my thoughts as I drove toward my childhood home of Parsons, Kansas, to put holiday flowers on her grave. The very first flowers placed there was shortly after her death on August 3, 2000. I'm glad I didn't know in my earlier life about the seven year struggle with Alzheimer's disease that would first rob her of her identity and then slowly take her life at the age of 91.

Leaving our farm near Miami, Oklahoma, on Spring River, the terrain slowly changes from the gently sloping hills of Northeast Oklahoma to the grassy flatlands of Kansas. In Kansas, one can drive for miles and not be bothered by abrupt changes in the terrain, except for an occasional wide spot in the road and towns with names like Columbus, Chetopa, and Oswego. In the stifling hot summer, cows behind barbed wire fences plod though pastures dotted with wild flowers or lie in the somewhat cooler shade of a century old oak. Nothing really protects beast or man from the scorching heat and unbearable humidity of a Midwest summer. Unceremoniously, farmers plow and harvest the fertile fields and gamble against draught and flood. Gargantuan patches of golden wheat seem to stretch out forever and intermingle with a great variety of other produce like corn and alfalfa.

Parsons comes into view, and I pass my childhood home—a large white frame house on Kennedy Street. The street was not named for JFK but for an early physician when the town first came into being. Parsons was named for Judge Levi Parsons, the first president of the M-K-T (Missouri, Kansas, and Texas) or Katy railroad, the reason for the founding of the town.[2] Even the name of the company has changed because it was bought up by the Union Pacific railroad in recent years. My dad worked as a locomotive engineer and was on the road a great deal running passenger trains. We all used to sit on the spacious front porch of that old house—my mom, my two brothers Jon, Carlos, and I. We ate buttered popcorn, real butter, or simply paused to watch the cars and the world go by. The big tree in the front yard has been cut down where my brother Jon perched for a strategic view of the neighborhood.

Mom was always at home waiting for us after our three block walk home from school. She often asked, "How did everything go at school today? Did you learn anything?" Sounding like we had just been released from prison, we usually replied, "No." It was the 1950's, and the boogie man was mostly in our imaginations. We could walk another three blocks to our grandparents' house without much worry. Of course, we would pass friendly neighbors, who all knew us and each other, as well as an aunt and uncle, Claude and my mother's oldest sister Bernie.

The neighborhood kids gathered to play in our rickety

old garage that had stalls where coal had been stored in an earlier era. In one of the three sections, which was no longer in use, my brothers built a ceiling with a trap door so that we could stand on top to play. It also served as a meeting place for the secret club house and a stepping stone onto which we climbed through a crawl space and hoisted ourselves up to the roof. At first neighbors called to snitch on us. Mom would say in a matter-of-fact tone, "If they figured out how to get up there, they can figure out how to get down."

We had a friendly war going on with our cousins who lived down the alley, the children of Mom's youngest sister Maxine and her husband Dan. When the cousins came onto our turf, we dropped small paper sacks of water on their unsuspecting heads, until Mom caught us. I didn't get in on everything my brothers and the boy cousins did, and so I'm sure that Eddie and Larry got their revenge.

One day my brothers suggested that we all jump from the garage roof, and they graciously let me go first. I was the youngest of the family and the only girl, and so I would pretty much go along with whatever they did so I wouldn't be called a sissy. Fortunately, I was limber, acrobatic, and knew how to take a fall. I jumped, landed with bent springy knees, and rolled over and over in the dust and gravel. The boys never did jump.

Mom never let us get out of her sight for too long but wasn't breathing down our necks either. The first time I complained to her that the boys were playing too rough, she said, "Don't play with them if you can't take it." When she witnessed my jump from her back porch view, she just yelled, "Don't break your leg before the dance recital. Your costumes are already paid for." She called me her tomboy ballerina. She gave us a great deal of attention and guidance, but she also let us somewhat suffer from the consequences of our own behavior and occasional stupidity.

The house was old even then. Dad thought it was reasonable to save a major part of the money first before buying a new house, which he did in 1962, the start of my senior year in high school. He had the Depression-era thinking, which is totally foreign to some people today. Mom's philosophy was that we couldn't hurt the old house that much, and so we pretty much had free reign to play out whatever our imaginations decreed. She was a bit of a kid herself, especially when my more serious father was out on passenger runs.

Although Mom had never been the greatest cook, she was always cooking up some fun. On rainy days, we spread out a tablecloth for a picnic on our living room floor, or we enjoyed campouts on the wagon trail in a tent made with a card table covered by an old wool blanket. We sat around an imaginary camp fire and told ghost stories. In the middle of one of Mom's most dramatic presentations about a ghost that walked the house at midnight, a young guest got so scared he had to call his mother and cried to go home early. We three kids were used to an atmosphere charged with adventure. We thought it was normal. She gave us the gift of imagination and the feeling that it was possible to accomplish almost anything. Recently, my brother Jon said that the best thing about that old house on Kennedy street was Mom.

The plastered ceiling had partially fallen in the dining room. Often the door knob on the front door came off in our hands, but we dutifully put it back. It didn't matter too much since we hardly ever locked our doors anyway. The whoosh of running water in the toilet in the main bathroom filled our ears so often that we hardly noticed it. When one of us tried to fix it, the lid on the flush tank made a loud thud when it crashed onto the old wood floor, breaking into two pieces.

Dad was a good engineer but a lousy repair man. When Dad announced that it was time to paint the bathroom, I offered to paint the low part. He let the paint slip out of the roller pan, and it drizzled down my back. I accidentally got in the way of a flying plumbing wrench on another occasion as I watched him too closely over his shoulder. I finally wised up and quit offering to help him. It was just easier to let things go—and less dangerous.

After we found a rusty old set of my grandfather's golf clubs, we were the only kids in town who could play miniature golf in our basement because of the holes in the concrete. Mom's philosophy about our house was that if nobody liked it, they didn't have to come. That taught me never to judge people by their homes or other possessions. In spite of its rundown condition, children in the neighborhood loved to gather there. In our teenage years, our friends liked to "hang out" at our house because Mom was fun—like one of us.

At the Tri-City airport, just outside Parsons, I can still see the tears coming out from under her dark sunglasses the day I left for Houston to become a flight attendant after college. The day I married my first husband Rob, she held the train of my long white dress and negotiated mud puddles, like a soldier on an obstacle course, all the way into church.

Garth Brooks was certainly right when he sang that song. Would any of us continue to live life to the fullest if we knew what was ahead?

> *Our lives are better left to chance*
> *I could have missed the pain*
> *But I'd have had to miss the dance.*[3]

Seeds of Faith

Childhood memories from church attendance include the dry vanilla wafers and tart orange juice I choked down at Sunday school, a missionary who reported that he had actually seen bananas growing on a tree, memorizing the books of the Old Testament in a song, and the day my brother Jon was baptized. Colors were ablaze in the stained glass windows, and the flicker of candlelight flirted with its own reflection into the baptismal pool. Mom had dutifully ironed the casual shirt and jeans that my brother was to be baptized in, sent his best suit to the cleaners, and then spent extra time starching and pressing the dress shirt he was to wear with his suit at the end of the service. The children came out one by one. My mother's blue eyes popped when she saw Jon walking toward the water wearing his Sunday suit. When the children came back for the rest of the service, all he had to wear were his jeans and old shirt. Mom wasn't angry but asked him why he had worn his good suit in the water, to which he replied, "Nothing is too good for the Lord."

When I was around twelve, we all joined St. John's Episcopal Church because Mom wanted Dad to go to church with us. Both churches were so different that I grew up realizing that there was something good in all denominations. I still hold that belief. Even though I mention things that happened to me in church, it is not the purpose of this book to promote any one Christian denomination. This is the story of my experience. I really do believe that we are more alike than we are different, and we all have common life experiences. Dealing with a beloved aging parent is universal and definitely a major one.

It's been several months since my mother Margaret passed on. I used to say passed away or when I felt really truthful, I would simply say that a person had died. Now I know, not just in my head but in my heart, that she truly passed on to something better than any of us can ever imagine. As a child, I was told that good people went to heaven, and I was sure, even then, that if anyone would go to heaven, my mother would. Not that she was saintly, but because of her great love for the Lord.

When I would tell friends and relatives about my wanting to write this book, they would often ask a similar question. "Do you want people to know that if you can make it through this struggle, so can they?" Yes, I guess, but it's much more than that. Along with the anguish of watching a family member lose who they are, there can also be an opportunity for learning major life lessons, personal growth, and in my case—salvation. I don't pretend to have all the answers. I just wanted to share what happened to me. I wanted people who are going through any trying experience to know that when you think that life has dealt you the worst, sometimes there are gifts in disguise. In this case, her gift to me was my salvation. What better gift could a mother give to a child?

Like some people, I went off to college and lost my faith somewhere along the way. It stayed lost for over thirty years until my mother started showing signs of Alzheimer's disease around seven years ago. Before this life-changing event, I thought I was pretty much in control of my life. My parents provided me with a good education. I had just remarried after my first husband Rob died of a massive heart attack at the age of 42. In a time of high divorce rates, I feel fortunate to have had two good marriages, not perfect but good.

Arley and I had just built a new house in a small resort town named Grove in the northeastern corner of Oklahoma. I had accomplished many of the career and personal goals I had worked so hard to achieve. Then life changed.

In June of 1994, I took Mom to the Dallas area to see her great-grandson Erik, who was approximately two months old at the time, as well as her oldest great-grandson Dustin, who described her as his "bestest buddy." She had a great love for children and the attraction was mutual. The drive home from Texas to Miami, Oklahoma, my home at that time, was approximately six hours, not counting rest stops. Driving back, the longer I was on the road, the worse I felt. We got as far as Eufaula, Oklahoma, which is a little over half way home and stopped to have lunch. All I felt like eating was the vegetable soup, but when the waitress brought it to me, I couldn't even eat that. Yes, I was getting the flu.

Mom was in the age group of remembering the Model T, and she, as well as her two sisters, Maxine and Bernie, had never learned to drive. For safety reasons, we just got a motel, and then I called my husband Arley when I knew he would be home from work. I didn't reach him until around six PM, and so we agreed that he would just wait and pick us up in the morning since it was about a three hour drive; besides, we had already settled into the motel room. Being the considerate and resourceful husband that he is, he came to pick us up the next day with his Chevy Blazer and a flatbed trailer and hauled the Honda home. By that time, I was definitely too sick to drive.

In that small motel room the night before, I began to notice that there was something different about my mother. We are all so busy with our lives that it is easy not to notice certain signs, even when it is someone so close to us as a parent. In this case, I was forced to observe her over a longer period of time without any distractions. Being ill and unable to move far from my bed, I could either watch her or TV. She had her suitcase on the table by the TV set, as in most motels, and so I was able to see both her and the TV set with ease. It is not unusual for a person to go through their suitcase several times to make sure they have what they need and didn't leave anything really important behind. In this instance, she rummaged through her suitcase for more than half an hour, turning and examining her clothes over and over again. This was my first realization that something was very wrong.

It became more and more apparent as time went on that my mother had severe short term memory loss. The circumstances were far beyond my control and problem solving abilities. It changed every fiber of my being. This was the beginning of a long journey that would bring me down so far into the abyss that I thought I would never find my way out. At the same time, it was an experience that brought me back to the Lord and helped me understand why my mother had such a great love for Jesus. Growing up, I would see her pass a picture of the Lord and touch it in a loving way with a smile and eyes filled with affection and adoration. When I quit going to church, she never preached at me or tried to stuff religion down my throat, but the seeds of faith she planted in my childhood came back at a crucial time to help me through the most trying period in my life—seeing her mind and eventually her body deteriorate.

As a child, I would often hear Mom say, "I sure hope I don't get that Old-Timer's disease." Almost all the women on my mom's side of the family lived very long lives—into their mid-eighties and mid-nineties. Unfortunately, almost all of them suffered dementia the last years of their lives. The other thing she dreaded was that someday she would be put in a nursing home. Both things eventually came true.

Although I now know how wrong it was, I wondered why a just and loving God would take the person I loved the most and make me watch her deteriorate over a long and agonizing period of time. I had heard people say things like: "The six months or the two years that my parent was ill was the worst time of my life." Even early in my experience, I knew the average course of AD was around seven years. As time went by, I compared it to the Chinese water torture where water is dripped on a person's forehead slowly and repeatedly until it drives them insane. It was like a duck pecking me to death. It was slow and insidious. It was like something tearing small pieces from my heart slowly and continuously. It was knowing my destiny and my mother's destiny and not being able to do a thing about it.

Once when I must have looked frustrated because I had to keep answering the same questions over and over again, a sad expression came on her face as she said, "I asked that before, didn't I?" It was then I decided I would try my hardest to remain patient no matter how many times she repeated the same thing. This was to be more difficult than I imagined. Ever since I could remember, Mom was always quick to laugh at her own mistakes and make a joke of her shortcomings. One day I said, "Mom, you don't laugh at your mistakes anymore." She replied, "You don't laugh either."

About a week before Christmas of 1994, a short time before Mom moved into an assisted living facility near my home, I asked her if she would like to come to Miami, Oklahoma, to spend Christmas day with us. Sometimes, she went to the home of one of my two brothers and their families. Basically, I just wanted to make sure she had somewhere to go for the holidays. She said that she was going to one of my brothers' homes, or they were coming to her apartment in Parsons. She couldn't remember which one. I just figured that she just hadn't made up her mind yet.

On Christmas Eve day, I called her again, and she said that she thought that one of my brothers was coming to pick her up soon. Realizing her confusion, Arley and I rearranged our Christmas schedule and quickly headed to Parsons. We needed to get back to make preparations for his two sons Randy and Mike, Mike's son Jeremiah, our daughter-in-law Jennifer, and Arley's mother Ruth. We were getting the idea that she might not have a place to go for Christmas because she had probably told both my brothers the same thing she told us, which was that she thought someone else had invited her. We finally talked her into coming home with us.

When we got to her apartment in Parsons that night, she looked so small and so lonely watching the Christmas Eve services on TV. She bravely sat in her white sweat shirt with a glittering poinsettia print around her shoulders. She was so confused that she couldn't remember what her Christmas plans had been. She was just waiting for one of us three kids to come. All of us thought she was going somewhere else. At first she refused to go home with Arley and me because she thought one of my brothers might come. After calling both brothers out-of-state, we finally convinced her that she should come celebrate at our house.

At this time, I began to have a slight understanding about what Mary must have felt giving birth to the Savior of the world yet knowing His destiny. She gave birth, watched Him grow up, saw Him mature in His ministry, and then had to watch Him die on the cross for our sins. Although she understood her great role, she was still subject to the suffering any mother would feel at knowing the destiny of her loved one and not be able to change the course of events.

Of course, I knew very well what would happen after Mom was diagnosed, but until that time I'm glad our family had just enjoyed life together—not knowing how it would all end for her. After saying this, knowledge of the progression of the disease is very important in keeping one's sanity. I solicited extensive material from the Alzheimer's Association. I questioned the professionals who dealt on a daily basis with people who suffered from AD or other dementia. With late life dementia so prevalent in my own family, I certainly plan to take advantage of any advances in medical science as soon as it available. Currently, several medications improve short term memory and others help slow down the progression of AD, but there is no prevention and no known cure as yet. Like many sons and daughters of dementia patients, I desperately pray that a cure will come in my lifetime.

Although being around nursing homes can be extremely depressing at times, it can certainly make one grateful. Toward the end of Mom's illness, I might be down about something at work, but after a visit to the nursing home and seeing people in a failing condition, I was sad, but at the same time, I would be glad to be able to walk, talk, and have a brain that functioned reasonably well. Aging and death certainly puts life and one's spiritual priorities into perspective.

Signs of Decline

Signs of short term memory loss of a friend or family member don't become apparent all at once. It slowly seeps into one's consciousness. The first signs of confusion had become apparent to me in June of 1994 in that motel room on our way home from the Dallas area, but I know that there must have been signs before this I hadn't noticed until I searched my own memory. Most people wouldn't know the exact time period as I do, but I am grateful that the Lord arranged things to let me slowly know the truth so that I could prepare somewhat for what was ahead.

Looking back, my oldest brother Jon's wife Fran remembered how hard it was for Mom to make her last two afghans, which were wedding presents for Arley and me. She had been crocheting for years, but, according to my sister-in-law Fran, Mom had to ask her over and over again how to complete certain tasks. This would have been around 1989, shortly after Arley and I were married. She made an afghan for me in the Southwestern colors of cactus green, sand, and clay for our new house. Since Arley is an avid sportsman, she crocheted an afghan for him in camouflage colors. Knowing what a struggle it was for her to complete these last two afghans make them even more of a treasure to us now.

At that time, she was eighty-three and living independently in a senior citizen high-rise, Belmont Towers, in Parsons, Kansas, around an hour and ten minutes from my home. I would visit her at least once a month on Saturdays to make sure she had plenty of groceries and was well, but mostly because I loved her and really enjoyed her company. Her sister Maxine also lived on the same floor of the apartment building. Her daughter Marsha and her husband Jack would take Mom to the grocery store when they came to visit. They would check on my mom when they came, and I would check on Maxine. Another cousin Barbara and her friend Sandy would also include her in family activities.

As time went by, her confusion became more apparent at places like the grocery store and Wal-Mart because it would take her a great deal of time to make a decision. One time at Wal-Mart, I walked to another part of the store, came back in ten minutes, and she was still looking at the same section of food items. It was becoming more and more difficult for her to make a decision, even over simple things like deciding what groceries she needed to buy.

As the signs became more obvious, I started to visit every other Saturday. She had much more difficulty all the time keeping track of things. At the age of fifty-five, I have that problem now, but this was more often and much more pronounced. I helped her reorder when she lost her box of checks. We finally found them in a dresser drawer under a pile of underwear. I started balancing her bank statements after she cracked her wrist in a fall. Her math was still outstanding, but she would forget to add in interest and service charges. At that time, short term memory loss was mostly the culprit. Her mental functions were still pretty much intact. She would wake up every morning and do crossword puzzles and play solitaire, as she stated somewhat in jest, "To see if my hands and my mind are still working." Looking back, this tells me that she knew, even then, that her memory was failing her. Most people are able to cover up the dementia in the very early stages. This is the reason why it is so hard for friends and family members to detect the severity of the problem early on.

She would put things in odd places. She lost her billfold for over two weeks. When I was there, I spent a great deal of time trying to help her find it. I finally found it under a stack of dish towels in a kitchen drawer. This was the beginning of the fear and paranoia many AD patients start to exhibit because of their memory loss. They begin to hide things, and then because of the memory loss, they can't remember where they put it. Then they might reason, "Did someone steal it?"

The fear and paranoia took another form. Being a railroad engineer most of his life, my father was on the road much of my childhood. Mom was never afraid to be alone in that big old house on Kennedy Street. He would be gone as long as two weeks at a time. Now, Mom was afraid to sleep in a three room apartment with her sister on the same floor. Mom and Maxine would spend some of the day alone or visit each other in one apartment or the other. However, the last year Mom lived at Belmont Towers, she always spent the night with her sister. She was just too afraid to sleep in her apartment by herself.

Other things started to happen. Her concept of time changed. She had been treated for high blood pressure for over twenty years. One time when she ran out of her prescription, she waited until the next time I came for a visit, which was over a week and a half later. She lived downtown only a few blocks from the pharmacy. The pharmacy also delivered, but it never occurred to her to do it the way she had in the past. I got her prescription filled as quickly as I could, and fortunately, there were no physical problems as a result.

I was now convinced that she could no longer live alone. The only reason she had remained somewhat independent was because of the elderly services of the high rise and her sister living on the same floor. She and Maxine were together almost constantly; it was almost like they were living together. I knew it was getting to be time to move her close to me, but I wanted them to stay together as long as possible. I had to work and knew that I couldn't give her anywhere near the time they spent together. As it was, they could enjoy each other's company all day.

At every visit, I tried to be alert to any changes in her living conditions. I began to check to see how long the lunch meat and other perishable food items had been in the refrigerator. I was afraid that she would become ill from food that should have been discarded because she was no longer able to remember how long it had been there. Again, Maxine would check on that also. Sometimes she would forget to eat altogether, and I was beginning to suspect that she was snacking on sweets as much as she was eating a regular meal. It was frustrating to me because I knew that there was no way I could know for sure. I knew even if I asked her, she probably wouldn't have remembered anyway. Because of this, I tried to get her to eat at least one meal at noon from Meals on Wheels. This way I would be assured that she ate at least one balanced meal a day.

Until one has tried to deal with someone afflicted with short term memory loss, it is hard to comprehend the extent to which it affects everyday life. Much to their embarrassment, I have even caught people who worked daily with AD patients ask: "Don't you remember? I told you that this morning." With my limited experience, I thought that eating lunch through Meals on Wheels was a great idea because all she had to do was to go downstairs and get her food. This didn't work either. She would either forget to go or forget she was supposed to go. I thought of putting up a sign to remind her, but then I figured she would either forget the sign was there, or if she did read it, she would forget what it said in a matter of minutes.

When I told the manager of the senior high rise about the problem, she suggested that someone on the same floor could come to her door and remind her that it was lunchtime. When I told Mom about the offer to help, she said, "I really don't like being around a bunch of old people." She was around eighty-four at the time. She didn't feel old. At the age of seventy-six, she had gone with me on a youth tour to Europe, led by one of the teachers in Jay, Oklahoma, where I was teaching at the time. Mom wasn't being uncooperative. She simply didn't know that her daily routine was coming unraveled.

She got into the senior van one day to go to the doctor and forgot where she was supposed to go. The van driver saw an appointment card in her hand and took her to the clinic. Now, it seemed she could no longer live alone, even with her sister's help. Maxine was a couple of years younger but was aging and had her own health problems. As much as she loved her sister, Maxine was starting to be weary of dealing with Mom's memory loss, which resulted in confusion and constant repetition. As with most AD patients in the early stages, she asked the same questions over and over again. Anyway, it wasn't her sister's responsibility to cope with it—it was mine. The living arrangement was no longer working. It was then our family decided to move her. We found Seneca Home Place in Seneca, Missouri, about 20 miles from my home in Miami.

Awakened

When it came time for Mom to move closer to me, I looked all over surrounding towns such as Grove, Afton, and Welch, Oklahoma, for an assisted living facility. She was not yet at a stage that she needed nursing home care, but she could no longer live independently. Several places I visited were beautiful but also very expensive. She received a railroad retirement pension because of my father's employment, but since he died before he was fully retired, it still wasn't enough to pay for the more luxurious assisted living places. This was the first time in my life I tried to make something work out that was extremely important to me and just couldn't.

A few of the less expensive facilities were in old run-down houses. The furniture was old and worn; the décor was drab and depressing. The number of workers was usually minimal, and there was little time to give each resident individual attention. As far as I could see, there were few activities for a physically healthy person like my mother. Additional residents came in for adult day care. Some rooms were shared by three people with very little living space. Even though I knew she couldn't afford a private room, I wanted her to have as many belongings around as possible to comfort her. I wanted her to live in a stable home-like environment that wasn't crowded. She had lived alone for so many years that I knew she needed a certain amount of privacy. Most of all,

I loved my mother so much and couldn't bear to see her live in what she and I would consider a dump.

I still felt guilty at times that I couldn't take care of her in my own home, but she was afraid to stay out in the country alone, and I was within five years of retiring from teaching. I really didn't want to quit my job so close to retirement. I knew that the progression of AD could last anywhere from two to twenty years with an average of seven years. If I did quit my job, I might have been forced to start teaching again in my late fifties or early sixties, even if I could get a job at that age. If a school district has a choice of hiring a good teacher with five years experience as opposed to twenty years experience, the school board will most likely hire the teacher who is much lower on the salary schedule. With tight school budgets, that savings can be readily used in other areas. From my point of view, dealing with teenagers at that age was too difficult for me even to imagine. I also needed to make it to retirement to secure my financial future.

My brothers would have taken care of her, too, but they both traveled extensively. The point is that I really wanted to move her close to me, but I couldn't find a nice place in Oklahoma that she could afford. Just as I was as stumped as I had ever been in my life, I cried out in my mind, "God, you have to help me!" It was more out of frustration than a real prayer, but help me He did.

Being close to the Kansas, Arkansas, and Missouri state line, we lived in what the locals call the Four State area. Arley worked in Neosho, Missouri, which is about a forty minute drive. The very next day, he came home and said that someone was opening a new assisted living facility in Seneca, Missouri, only about a twenty minute drive from Miami. I thought it would probably be too expensive, but I checked it out anyway. I found that I was a few hundred dollars short a month. In Missouri, Family Services will give seniors a small grant to help pay for assisted living to keep them out of the nursing homes as long as possible because of the greater expense to the state.

The Lord had answered my prayer in a big way. Dan Dareing, pastor of Elk River Baptist Church where I now attend, says that Jesus is on the other side of the door, but the door knob is on our side. By just opening the door a crack, His love came pouring through. At this stage I was amazed but still not totally convinced. Was this just a coincidence, I thought? Brother Dan also says, "God always gives us the choice to believe or not to believe."

In the Bible we are taught to believe in the unseen and not ask for signs and wonders. In Matthew 4:1–7 Jesus was led into the wilderness and was tempted by the devil. The devil also took him to the holy city to stand on the highest point of the temple. The devil told Jesus to throw himself down because, according to scripture, the angels would surely catch his fall. Jesus answered him, "Do not put the Lord your God to the test."

Even at that time, deep in my mind, I knew that people shouldn't make demands of God or ask for signs. In spite of this, one night in bed I said to myself, "God, if you're up there, please let me know." At the speed of light, a gentle hand touched my shoulder. Then I turned toward Arley to tell him what had happened. I told him that as soon as I asked God to let me know if He was up there, I felt you touch my shoulder. Arley replied, "You woke me up. I never touched your shoulder. I was asleep." Did Arley touch my shoulder? Was it Jesus? Again, I could choose to believe or not to believe.

Around the same time, I decided to visit two very good friends in Claremore, Oklahoma, Bob and Johanna. We had been friends since our early thirties, and our friendship has stayed in tact through many life changes. We "knew each other's warts," as Johanna put it, but all loved each other just the same.

We had often talked about spiritual experiences, and

these two had faith beyond my comprehension. Several years earlier, they had both quit very good jobs because Bob felt called to make rosaries. Not knowing if they would make enough money to keep their home, they both went into this home-based business on faith alone. Johanna did the business end but also expanded into selling other religious items. It had been a long struggle, but they not only didn't lose their home, the business has prospered into a comfortable living.

They are always very occupied at home with their business but are able to visit with me when I'm there. I just have to work around their schedule, and I offer to help at times. On a few occasions, I have helped them pack shipments for delivery. I have threatened more than once to put a card in the box to read: "Packed by a Protestant." The conversation would often turn to spirituality. I always found it refreshing that people of two different religious viewpoints could come together and find common ground. In the final analysis, all Christians love Jesus. On that particular visit, I decided to stay overnight to have a longer time to be with them. They asked if I would like to go to church with them the next morning. Since I had grown up from age twelve to twenty in the Episcopal church, I felt fairly comfortable in the Catholic church.

St. Cecilia's is a very beautiful and inspiring church in Claremore. As we sat in Sunday mass, a very definite voice came into my head, "What are you waiting for—a phone call?" It was like someone outside myself speaking to me. Could this be God, I thought? Some people have visions, some are slain in the Spirit and Moses had the burning bush. How could I get something weird like this? Was this God's equivalent to saying, "Must I get your attention with a ball bat?" Do you think God has a sense of humor? He must have. He created Robin Williams.

After mass I told Bob and Johanna about my message. I asked Johanna if she thought it was Jesus. She said, "By the look on your face, I'd say yes." I then asked her why He would speak to me in such a light-hearted way. She said, "He probably wanted to temper it with humor so it wouldn't scare you too much." If that's the case, I'm glad He did. That was enough to put me in orbit for a while.

After Mom's death several years later, I joined Elk River Baptist Church in Grove, Oklahoma, a community where Arley and I plan to retire. Brother Dan had a way of answering many of the questions I have had for so many years. In one of his sermons, he said that most new Christians want a bolt of lightening or something very dramatic to happen as a sign from God in order to believe. He went on to say that usually Jesus just speaks to us in a soft, still voice.

I wrote the following poem, *Collect Call*, to remember and to give thanks for this one-way whimsical conversation with the Lord:

Collect Call
(On Judgment Day)

God won't call
On the telephone.
Won't leave a message
If you're not home.
God tries to reach us
Each and every day.
Prayer is the answer.
The only way.
If He calls long distance,
What will you say
When He calls collect
For you on Judgment Day.

Get a pager
With your telephone.
Get beeped and buzzed

Till the cows come home.
But the call won't come
Unless you pray.
You can't put God "on hold"
Come Judgment Day.

The information highway
Is the place to speed.
The World Wide Web
Is fun to read.
Dust off the Bible.
That's all you need.
Get on-line with the Lord
To eternity.

Judith Ames David

A Moving Experience

Packing up and moving my mother from Parsons, Kansas, to Seneca, Missouri, was an experience I will never forget. It was late October of 1995. I had to find some way to get Mom to move closer to me and make her understand that it was best for her to do so. She had always taught us to be honest. One time I borrowed one of her library books, and about the time it was due, she became very worried that I wouldn't return it on time. I just said, "It's no big deal if it's late. It's just a few cents a day fine." She retorted, "I've never had an overdue library book, and I don't plan on starting this late in life." Now, I was in a position to really stretch the truth to someone who was so honest and conscientious that she had always turned in library books on time and would feel terrible if she didn't. I hated being less than honest with her, but I really loved my mother and just wanted to protect her.

I do remember one time when I was in the third grade when she stretched the truth a great deal because of her love for me. Mom had always wanted to take dancing lessons as a child but was forced to play the piano. Yes, you guessed it; I started taking dancing lessons at the age of four. I took tap, acrobatics, ballet, jazz, and eventually put on toe shoes and went on point. Toe dancing was not my calling. A bird dog went on point better than I did. I did like everything else though. This particular year, my dance teacher, Nell Ferguson, decided to combine my abilities in tap dancing and acrobatics.

Being an acrobatic tap dancer or a tap dancing acrobat was no small accomplishment for a third grader. I was not a newcomer to the stage having twice danced in the Nell Ferguson Review at the Parsons Municipal Building stage, the intermission at the local picture show, and the Old Soldier's Reunion and Bean Supper in Erie, Kansas. Now, my dancing teacher had selected me to appear on television. (Back in those days, people were so fascinated with TV that they would watch anything.) The KOAM Channel 7 Fun Club in Pittsburg, Kansas, was maybe, some said, a stepping stone to *Ted Mack's Original Amateur Hour.* The Old Forty-Niner introduced my act while Mom gave me a good luck wink, and then put *By the Light of the Silvery Moon* on the portable phonograph.

I tap danced like machine gun fire, catapulted into cartwheels and splits, shuffled and kicked into a backbend—raising right arm/left leg then left arm/right leg. It was a contest. The contestant receiving the most post cards, or votes, would be the winner. Later on at home, Mom wrote out, signed, and mailed cards from cousins, aunts, uncles—living and deceased—from California to Washington, D. C., saying things like, "I'm sure if Uncle Ed were still alive, he would vote for you." In spite of her efforts, the first place prize, a gold wrist watch, went to a sister singing act from Coffeyville, Kansas. I won a chartreuse leopard TV lamp for second place. The two sisters must have had more relatives, more post cards, or a more determined mother.

Now it was my turn to twist the truth. I wasn't the perfect child or teenager, but I had always tried to stay on her good side. I didn't obey her out of fear as much as love and not wanting to disappoint her. I tried to explain to her that she needed to move closer to me because of her memory loss. She was convinced that she could still live on her own but welcomed the chance to live closer to one of her children.

It is so heart-breaking for the family members because there is no way you can explain to someone who has memory loss that this problem is interfering with their lives in a significant way. Even if you do convince them, they won't remember it in five minutes anyway.

After explaining it over and over again, I finally told her that if she didn't like her new place, she could move back to her apartment in Parsons. She cheerfully agreed, but I knew all the time there would be no going back. The last thing in the world I wanted to do was to be deceitful, but I felt I had no choice. At this point there was no way she could fully comprehend the situation. It really hurt, but I had to face the reality that if she stayed there, she could run out of medication, eat tainted lunch meat, or get lost walking to town.

She liked to save almost everything people gave her—cards, gifts, souvenirs. Although looking through the past with her was fun, I knew that she would be moving from a three room apartment to sharing a room with another lady. It became more apparent as the day went on that she didn't want to throw anything away. I could understand why she didn't want to throw away things like family photo albums and pictures that the grandchildren had drawn and lovingly given to her. There were other items, however, I failed to understand. I know that someone in the family at one time or another had given her mylar balloons for birthdays, Mother's Day, and other special occasions. I had probably given her a few. She didn't know who gave her what, but she insisted on keeping a stack of now very flat mylar balloons. This is just one example of the many treasures she refused to relinquish.

I finally had to wait until she went to bed. I slept with her that night so that she would go to sleep, and I could sort through the boxes later. Because of her memory loss, she kept talking to me and told me good night five or six times.

She would say, "Good night, honey. It sure is great having you here."

"It's great being here, Mom. Good night."
"Is there anything I could get you?"
"No, Mom, I'm just fine. See you in the morning."
"Do you have enough blankets?"
"Yes, I'm very comfortable."
"Do you want anything to drink? We could pop some popcorn if you're hungry."
"No, I'm not hungry, but I'm a little tired."
"Well, you had better get some sleep then."
"Okay, Mom. Good night."
"Good night, sweetheart. Can I get you anything before you go to sleep?"

I hated to do it, but I finally pretended I was asleep so that she would quit asking questions. Then I got up around 2:00 AM and started throwing things away down the chute in the hallway as fast as I could if it had no real value. I put sentimental things in her sister Maxine's apartment to divide among us three children later.

The next day, Arley came in our pickup to move her out of her apartment in Parsons while my brother Carlos and his daughter Carla came to help also. What we couldn't get into her new room I stored in our old rent house on the farm. At first she wondered where certain items were, and I told her they were in storage. Eventually, thank the Lord, she forgot all about them. At times she would say, "Do I still have my apartment in Parsons?" I would tell her that she didn't but could move back if she didn't like Seneca. I kept reminding her that Seneca was only about twenty minutes from our house and that seemed to satisfy her for a while. I had to keep stalling her until she finally made an adjustment to her new place. I felt so awful having to mislead her. All the time I knew that the move was permanent. Like I said, I felt like I didn't have any choice but to say what I did to keep her from being agitated and more confused.

One of the teachers at Miami High School where I taught at that time had experience in dealing with dementia in a family member. He thought the hardest part was during the early stages. They realize that something is wrong, but they can't do anything about it. As a person slips deeper into dementia, they are not as conscious of their mistakes and are, therefore, less embarrassed. In later stages, balanced medication helps control the agitation and confusion. After Mom's mind dove deeper into the disease, she went back to Parsons to Belmont Towers to visit her sister. She recognized her sister but didn't remember having lived in that building although it had been her home for over thirteen years.

During that time, she still seemed to be very normal in her day to day conversation. She could remember back twenty years ago but had a difficult time telling you what had happened even an hour ago. Although she lived at Seneca Home Place for two years, she never could remember which door was to the closet and which door was to the bathroom until she opened it. She got along very well with her roommate Alma, and her stay there was very pleasant. They laughed and joked and had a great time. Although I didn't fully comprehend it at the time, the Lord had answered my prayers in a very big way.

Shells

While picking up shells on the beach one day,
I found a fragment of what must have been
a magnificent conch . . .
a remnant of a masterpiece.
Holding it gently, I tried to imagine
the part as a whole
it was at its best, before it was
broken by time and the churning sea.
It must have been an elegant creature,
a prime of its species.
I thought of my mother
who was, before she was broken by time and
   degenerative disease,
a prime example of her species.
Those of us who remember the bright, gracious
   lovely lady
that she was at her best
are grateful when you,
who know only the remaining fragment
of herself,
handle her gently
as a once magnificent shell.[4]

Phyllis Young

The Fragment of a Shell

A short time after Mom began her decline into AD, I found this beautiful poem, "Shells," in the Oklahoma Chapter of the Alzheimer's Association newsletter. It precisely put into words how I felt about turning the care of my mother over to strangers who had not known what I considered "the real Mom." I carried this poem in the glove compartment of my car until after her death. It was a great comfort to me knowing that someone else knew exactly how I felt.

She lived at Seneca Home Place for two years and was happy with the pretty new facility, the caring staff, and her roommate Alma. Alma was a retired high school teacher and didn't mind answering the same questions over and over again. As a matter of fact, I think it made her feel useful. I was grateful to God for their friendship. It seemed to benefit both of them because she was a guide to Mom, and, in turn, Mom kept her laughing.

Predictably, the two years she spent there continued the slow but steady decline of her mental functioning. As Mom became more easily confused, the role reversal between us was more profound. Once she even questioned, "Are you my mother or am I your mother?" As I look back, one of my biggest losses was that I no longer had a mother to confide in. In addition, it was always a challenge to direct her without sounding like I was her boss. I still wanted to regard her as my mother. It wasn't always easy. I found myself playing some of the games with her that she had played with me as a child. To get her to go down the long hallway to dinner, we would walk in cadence arm in arm laughing when we missed the beat or landed on the wrong foot.

I LEFT, I LEFT
I LEFT my wife and 45 kids
due to starvation
without any gingerbread.
Think I did RIGHT?

During her stay in Seneca, Mom had more good days than bad days. It seemed to me that her bad days were sometimes a predictor of the way she would be in the next stage. The dreaded day finally came right around Christmas of 1996. At the beginning of one visit, I couldn't find Mom in her room or anywhere else in the facility. Then I saw her standing outside the back door for no apparent reason. When I mentioned this to one of the aides, she said that they didn't want to tell me until after Christmas because they didn't want to spoil the holidays for me, but this wandering had started to become a pattern. They had been watching her closely for the past two weeks. Even though there was a very large front lawn with a lengthy driveway in front of the facility, it perched on the corner where two busy highways intersected—Hwy 43 and 60.

She and her roommate Alma loved to look out the window or sit on the patio to watch the cars and semis go by. Seneca calls itself "the little border town" because it is in Missouri but on the Oklahoma border. Because of this, many trucks bypass the weigh stations at the state line by dipping down to Hwy 60 to get across the state line at that location. Crosses have been placed on at least two corners of the intersection indicating the loss of loved ones. Apparently, Mom had walked to the end of the long driveway to wait for her parents to pick her up. She was around eighty-seven at the time, and her parents had been dead for over forty years. It was obvious that she needed to move to a facility with more security where she couldn't wander off to the busy highway or get lost in the woods in back.

Due to this change in circumstances, our family made the decision to move her to a nursing home facility around fifteen minutes from Seneca. Because of the move to Medicalodge in Neosho, I was back in the business of figuring out what to do with the belongings from Seneca Home Place that wouldn't fit into her room at the nursing home. I had already thrown away, given away, or stored many of her possessions. Now, it was time to do it again. She didn't have many things of material worth, but it was still hard because of all the sentimental value attached to the belongings that remained. I could see myself in that position some day, having someone else making decisions about which one of my possessions I would keep and which would be stored or discarded into the trash.

The first day I took Mom to Medicalodge was easily one of the worst days in my life. I knew how she must have felt when she dropped me off at kindergarten for the first time. This was different, though. Instead of launching me on my educational career, I knew that this was just the opposite, graduating her into the final stage of her life. I think that this is why losing a parent or loved one this way is so devastating. They become a child who needs special protection and care. Because of the dementia, they are so dependent, and losing them is somewhat like losing a child. It broke my heart when she said, "Am I living here? What's wrong with these people?" I knew how she would feel if her "old self" could see her in this condition. She had seen firsthand the effects of dementia on several of her family members, and now her worst nightmare had come true. She was not only in a nursing home but in the Alzheimer's unit. I was so upset that I had to leave the nursing home for a while, go to the car to cry, and then come back later. It was too much reality to comprehend all at once because I knew that soon she would be exhibiting some of the same behavior that she even now considered odd.

I had no experience in dealing with a nursing home, which was pretty obvious by the amount of material possessions I tried to put in a room shared with another resident. Because of my selfish encroachment of territory, which I labeled "just doing my best for Mom," I soon met up with the nursing home administrator Evelyn Hottinger. I felt guilty about taking even more possessions away from Mom, and so I stuffed as much as possible on her side of the room. Her side had the window, the best side. The other side had the bathroom entrance, the sink, and the closets. I didn't understand that half of the wall in front of Mom's bed also belonged to the roommate since that side of the room had so little space in comparison. When all of this was taking place, I was only fifty-two at the time. Mom was thirty-seven when I was born, and so I was facing this situation much earlier than most people. Her first roommate was very aggressive and hostile, and so I asked for a different roommate. When Evelyn came into her room, she said, "I have worked in nursing homes all my adult life and have never seen so much stuff in one room."

I thought the room looked as bright and cozy as possible, considering the little space I had to work with. Evelyn and I were not fast friends. It took me some time to realize that life in a nursing home was quite a bit different from life in an assisted living facility. Evelyn, of course, had to do what was best for all concerned. I was just trying to protect my mom and do everything I could to make her comfortable and happy. The art of compromise solved the problem, and at the time I didn't know that Evelyn would play such a significant role in helping me to deal with my mother's eventual decline and passing. Because of Evelyn's courage and strong leadership, I was confident that she understood that even though the residents in her charge were only a fragment of what they once were, they were still worthwhile human beings who deserved all the help and respect she and her staff could possibly give.

A Time of Loss

The onset of AD marks the beginning of a time of loss—mental, emotional, social, and then eventually physical. Mom was to live at Medicalodge three and a half years before her death from the complications of AD. It was during this time that the disease progressed toward its final stages. To understand the impact of the intellectual loss caused by AD or other dementia, one must try to imagine living in a world in which you have no memory of what happened one hour ago, a minute ago, and then eventually a few seconds ago. Mom knew who I was for about the first year at Medicalodge. For about another year, sometimes she knew it was me; sometimes I was her sister Maxine; and sometimes I was her mother. At that period of time, even when she didn't know me, she knew that I was someone she loved or at least I was someone with whom she should be familiar.

Even the loss of seemingly small things can have an unexpected impact. In our family we have always had a ritual for saying goodbye—especially when we knew we wouldn't be seeing each other for quite a while. Everyone would go to the driveway, give goodbye hugs and kisses, and then wave until the car was out of sight. The family members leaving in the car would wave back and continue honking until they could no longer see us. We must have had great separation anxiety.

As a child, I thought that everyone made a spectacle

of themselves on these occasions. Sometimes when a family member was slow in leaving because of all the parting remarks, we would end up waving for a longer period of time than usual. As a result, we would get creative with our waving and look like a referee calling a foul at a basketball game or give a tired wave with one elbow propped on the other arm like Granny did at the end of *The Beverly Hillbillies* TV show. As a matter of fact, we probably looked like the Beverly Hillbillies.

When Mom went to Medicalodge, this ritual couldn't continue unless an aide walked to the car with us. This was just too much to ask for the busy staff members. Finally, I just asked someone on the staff to distract her so that I could leave. I couldn't bear to see her follow me to the locked door and not understand why she couldn't go with me. I would tell her goodbye, and then someone would either engage her in conversation blocking her view of me so that I could get out the door undetected, or they would take her down the other hall allegedly to show her something interesting. I hated to have to trick her like that, but sometimes there is no choice when an explanation cannot be understood. It's funny how even simple rituals like saying goodbye have to change. Every time I left her at the nursing home, I cried or felt like crying. This was the profound realization of how much the continual loss of mental function can color all aspects of the life of an AD victim, as well as the lives of the people who love them.

Have you ever thought about the many things you couldn't do if you had short term memory loss? Yes, it is true that people with AD and other dementia can many times remember twenty years ago better than an hour ago. How does this affect daily life? It affects everything. Basically, if one can't remember what happened seconds before, one can no longer enjoy reading a book, watching movies, or many of the other activities we take for granted every day.

Mom had been an avid reader. She could still read the

words, but by the time she finished reading a page, she had no memory of what she had read. The same was true of a movie. To people with short term memory loss, there is no longer any story with which to identify. Eventually, they lose interest in these and many other activities. They can hold a limited conversation, but it is difficult to make new friends because one has to remember a certain number of facts about the other person to form a relationship. The memory loss seems to make time stand still. For this reason, it is difficult for an AD patient to adjust to change, especially a major move, but with God's help and the caring staff at Medicalodge, she eventually did adjust.

I remember one instance when the loss of familiar activities came crashing to my attention. On Palm Sunday of 1999, I went for a visit. Most people her age were not as active. When I arrived, she was usually asleep or up walking around talking to other residents and staff members. On this occasion, however, she was just lying in bed staring out the window. I asked her why she was still in bed, and she said, "There's nothing to do." It hit me how her loss of familiar activities had made such a great impact on her life. At this stage, even when she was around family or doing what she liked to do, it would all be forgotten in a matter of minutes or even seconds after the person had left.

It was all I could do to keep from crying, but the futility of the situation was that she wouldn't understand why I was upset, it would be difficult to explain it to her, and even if somehow I could, she wouldn't remember it anyway. All I could do was to try to make the best of the day. She had always enjoyed going for a ride in the car and getting ice cream. Sometimes AD can work to a family member's advantage. After an enjoyable afternoon, Mom forgot all about the depression earlier in the day.

On another visit, I walked toward her to greet her with a hug, and she said, "I just got to thinking. Why should I go look for my daughter if she never comes to visit me?" She thought that I had abandoned her, even though I had visited her quite often. When she couldn't remember the visits, what other conclusion could she draw? The daughter she remembered looked like the pictures on her dresser from ten years ago—not like the woman with the graying hair and glasses who stood in front of her with a shocked look on her face. Choking back tears, I finally said, "I am your daughter, and I come to visit you all the time, but you can't remember it." The futility of the situation is hard to comprehend. It is a lesson in humility and unconditional love—to continue to love someone deeply when they don't know to love you back.

If I had learned unconditional love from anyone, it would have been Mom. Except for Christ, she was the best example of someone who loved without limits. This was a great gift for we three kids to know that she would love us no matter what. Like all elderly people, AD patients have their good days and their bad days. After a while, I learned not to have any expectations of what the visit would bring. I was lucky because a majority of the time she liked to get out, but because she was in her eighties, some days she would simply be too tired. Many people her age are confined to bed or to a wheelchair, and so I was lucky that we could still go out in the car, and we did so until around six weeks before she died.

Her unusually healthy condition was a plus in most cases, but sometimes it could be a negative. Because she could still walk without any assistance, she could also wander off at any given time. In big stores like Wal-Mart, I had to watch her and keep her in view as one would any five-year-old.

The last year and a half or so, she didn't know who I was most of the time. She never completely lost her ability to speak, but it became more difficult all the time for her to form coherent sentences. And the wandering up and down the hall became more prevalent. I remember several times I would be talking to her in her room, and if I glanced away to look in a drawer or out the window, she would be gone.

This constant wandering, although it was good exercise, also caused her to deteriorate more rapidly the last year or so because at this time she also lost her appetite. The combination of being physically overactive and eating less caused her to lose a great deal of weight. If you have ever tried to feed a toddler when they didn't want to eat, you can understand how difficult it is to feed an uncooperative adult who has a diminished mental capacity. AD affects the brain in many ways. Maybe, the part of the brain that stimulates the appetite is affected, and sometimes they just forget to eat. At five feet two inches, she had weighed only about 110 pounds anyway, and so a loss of ten or fifteen pounds was significant.

Other physical loss included several falls, which usually caused mostly bruises and skin tears. Nursing homes are required to call when a resident has fallen, even if there are minor or no apparent injuries. After a while, my insides jumped every time the phone rang. Ironically, I wasn't even home to receive the phone call when she broke her hip. I was out shopping for groceries after work in Miami, about a forty minute drive from Neosho. I picked Medicalodge because it had the best AD unit, even though I wished that I could have found a good facility closer to my home. My husband Arley worked in Neosho, and so when I wasn't home, they phoned him at the plant. They had her somewhat sedated when I got to the Neosho hospital, and they were ready to transfer her to a larger hospital in Joplin, Missouri, fifteen minutes away.

Early in 2001, when the Reagan family announced on TV that the former president had broken his hip, it reminded me how physical injuries are further complicated by AD. Incredible as it may sound, Mom did not remember that she had broken her hip. She had once said to my brother Jon, "Why didn't someone tell me that I broke my hip?" Not knowing how to answer at first, he paused and said, "We all thought you knew."

It's hard to hold back a chuckle until one realizes the consequences. As I stated previously, she was extremely active for her age and loved to walk and socialize. It was a dangerous scenario because she wasn't reminded of her injury until she got up and started to walk. Once up, there was a great possibility that she would fall and break something else. That was a very frightening time for me and the staff at Medicalodge. She just couldn't understand why she had to stay in a wheelchair. Physical restraints are against the law and would have just made her more determined and agitated, plus the fact that they are inhumane. They did put a lap cushion that hooked on the sides of the wheelchair that helped give them time to reach for her if she tried to get up.

They placed her in front of the nurses' station to watch her during the day. She had a personal alarm hooked on the back of her collar, which she set off quite often. She eventually learned to get out of it. It's amazing what AD patients can do, despite their impaired mental functions. At this time they put up the side rails on her bed for safety at night. She soon learned how to slide down to the bottom of the bed and maneuver around the bottom of the rails. One night she got out of bed and held herself up by walking hand over hand against the wall. The nurse at the desk looked up in horror and saw Mom leaning against the door in the hall ready for her nightly stroll. This was the time I definitely had to put her in the hands of the Lord and ask that angels protect her day and night.

Physical therapy at Medicalodge did an excellent job in her rehabilitation, but the staff still struggled with the worry of her getting up without someone being there to support her until she was fully rehabilitated. Several weeks after her cast was taken off, Martha, the director of nursing, said, "Let's just see what happens when we let her get up." Staff was ready in case of a fall. To the surprise of all, Martha said that she simply got up and started walking with a slight limp. There was no stopping her. She had always had exceptional balance, and it really paid off in this case. When she was first injured, the doctor warned me that for many people her age, a broken hip was the beginning of the end. Many elderly people go to bed and never get up. Not my Mom. Dr. Hill eventually learned to shake his head and accept her determination, zest for life, and will to live. Even when the AD changed her intellectual functioning and physical condition, it never broke her spirit.

The hardest loss of all was the loss of self. The last two years when she didn't know me most of the time, I would sometimes feel that I was just visiting her body. It seemed like over the seven years or so that Mom suffered from AD, I would just get used to dealing with one aspect of the disease, when another set of circumstances presented new challenges. I now know why it is called "the long goodbye." The progression is very slow and painful for all involved. With God's help, I learned to endure and turn to Him for strength.

Tears, Prayers, and Learning to Cope

How does one cope with seeing a friend or family member deteriorate from AD or other related disorders? We all have a variety of trials in our lives. How we react to them says something about who we are, as well as who we will become. I started out being angry because I didn't think a loving and just God would let a person like my mother suffer a long and debilitating illness like AD. Gradually throughout those seven years, I grew spiritually. Because of the way she reacted to her illness, Mom was an inspiration to many people, especially to me. Even when she didn't know anyone in particular, she reached out to everyone like a child. She never lost her loving spirit. Even when her body and mind continued to lose function, her spirit was evident to the end.

Throughout this ordeal, I learned that I couldn't and didn't want to live the rest of my life without feeling God's love and guidance. I was literally brought to my knees and learned to depend on prayer to retain my sanity. What at first seemed the ultimate tragedy later became the catalyst for my own salvation. What has happened to my mother and my family on this earth isn't nearly as important as what will happen in the next life, and eternity is a long, long time. Prayer didn't take away all the pain of the long struggle, but it did give me comfort in order to face reality and continue to cope.

The other aspect of coping was the ability to be honest about my feelings and simply cry when I needed to. Sometimes, when the occasion was not appropriate, I would have to wait until later. But cry I did. Being sad and releasing the frustration with tears is a very appropriate response to a sad situation. Some people hold back tears for such a long period of time because they believe if they do start crying, they will never stop. One time I tested this theory and proved it false. Try it yourself. After a while, I was so exhausted that I couldn't cry anymore. I was so afraid that if I let my feelings out completely, I might go insane. The opposite is true. All I felt was a great sense of relief.

If one isn't honest about his or her own feelings, it will come out as something else—usually anger directed toward others. Many times when I felt tense about her situation or just life in general, I then realized I just needed to cry. This was the only way I could keep going back to visit my mother time after time. I wanted and needed to keep going back because I loved her so much, but I was able to keep going back because facing my feelings honestly and crying when necessary was the best release of frustration, as we all know.

I believe the reason that some people avoid seeing loved ones on a regular basis in a nursing home is because they don't want to deal with the pain. When I was studying for an MS degree in Counseling many years ago, I took a course entitled, *Death and Dying*. Strange as it may seem, it was one of the most valuable classes I have ever taken. One very important thing I learned was that dying isn't the worst thing that can happen to a person, but dying alone is. I was determined that my mother would not go through the deterioration of AD, or die, alone. Because of this decision, I learned more about my own aging and eventual death. I believe that it is important to let yourself feel your feelings and face the reality of your circumstances in order to grow spiritually.

I learned that one must accept his or her own death in order to appreciate how precious life is. Elisabeth Kubler-

Ross wrote a definitive book about the grieving process called *On Death and Dying*, which, among many other aspects of dealing with death, named the stages of grief—shock and denial, anger, bargaining, depression, and acceptance. She also talked about America being a denial society. We are no longer close to death as our ancestors were. Families in the past were often multi-generational, and the elderly died in the home with loved ones around, including small children. Now, families are flung far and wide. Because people are more mobile today, and many women find it necessary to work, the elderly are often cared for in nursing homes, and people often die in these nursing homes or in hospitals. Because death has become somewhat institutionalized, it is much easier for us to remove ourselves from it. We don't even see animals slaughtered on a farm for food. We just go to the grocery store and pick up neatly wrapped, sanitized and plasticized packages of meat. If we can't meet death on its terms with our family members, we will be unable to put our own aging and death into perspective. Kubler-Ross calls going through this process grief work. It is something that is necessary to heal and not let the pain control us. We must allow ourselves to go through the pain of loss or even anticipated loss to accept death and eventually get back to the business of life.[5]

With the slow progression of AD, I found that I had to grieve each new stage of deterioration. Because of the seven year time period, for me it wasn't just one big loss but a whole series of losses. Stress over a long period of time can be a killer if one doesn't find some way of releasing the tension. If you stuff your feelings under the carpet, you won't be able to see them, but they will still be there. Eventually, it will emerge as some other inappropriate emotion later, usually anger.

A staff member at Medicalodge once told me, "Don't get mad at the disease." In other words, if you can try to understand how AD manifests itself and progresses throughout the various stages, you won't take the negative actions of your loved one so personally. If your loved one is having a bad day and gets angry at you for no apparent reason, it still hurts, but it will be more understandable. I found that a certain amount of knowledge once my mother was diagnosed helped to take the sting out of many uncomfortable and sometimes painful situations.

Being a retired high school English teacher hardly qualifies me to give medical advice. This is why I turned to the professionals. The brain is affected by a disease that eventually alters behavior in a drastic way, but it has a physical basis. In the year or so that Mom was still able to live alone but on the same floor as her sister in senior housing, I obtained a vast amount of material from our local hospital, as well as the Alzheimer's Association. My nearest chapter was in Tulsa, Oklahoma. For more information on how they can help, call information for the chapter nearest you or find them online. There is a very helpful newsletter that comes in the mail, and you can get updates on all aspects of AD and other related disorders on the internet. You will never know what the professionals know, but basic knowledge of the disease will give you clues about what to expect as the disease progresses. It won't keep the deterioration from happening, and it won't keep you from having to endure the pain of witnessing it, but it will prepare you somewhat for what's ahead.

No matter what your lifestyle or circumstances are, you must maintain open communication with people who care about you. It is the only thing that will help you stay sane. If you don't have an understanding person to talk to on a regular basis, join a support group. The Alzheimer's Association has support groups, and there are groups associated with many hospitals and nursing homes. Ask around and you'll find one.

I think it is also important to be open and honest about your situation. Although I think it's not wise to "wear your heart on your sleeves," key people, especially if you work, need to know the situation. I had to miss work occasionally to take Mom to the doctor or help her in the hospital, and so my very understanding principal and caring school secretary knew more details than most.

During class one day, I was really depressed about dealing with my mother's AD. This time, instead of being impatient or in a bad mood but covering up my pain, I just told one of my classes how I was feeling about Mom. I didn't know if young people could even relate or care about this problem. My being honest about my feelings opened up a whole class discussion about AD because several teenagers in that class had a beloved grandparent who suffered from dementia. By my discussing how I felt, they could more readily understand what their parents were experiencing and perhaps be more patient with them. I knew that people my age and older were dealing with it, but I forgot that young members of the family were highly affected also.

Whenever Mom was in the hospital, I felt I needed to be there most of the time because an AD patient has trouble communicating with the medical staff. They are also more afraid because they don't know what is wrong with them or where they are. Constant reassurance from a loved one is helpful in the healing process. Other family members have also assisted in staying the night in the hospital to make sure her needs were met and to give her the security she needed.

As my mother progressed more into the disease, I found that I was able to help friends whose loved one was starting to show signs of memory loss. One of the most important things I had discovered was that you are of no help to your loved one if you lose your physical and/or mental health. It's not fair to the other people in your life if you let AD conquer your mind, body, and soul. I also knew that the last thing my mother would want was for her to be the cause of my downfall.

When Mom first started showing signs of short term

memory loss, I felt somewhat isolated in my struggle. Former President Ronald Reagan was diagnosed with AD shortly after my mother's memory started failing her. This really helped me to put things into perspective. I knew that my mother had been a capable and intelligent person before AD. After I learned that the former president was afflicted with it, it was a great reminder that this disease does not discriminate. It can even happen to the head of state of the most powerful country in the world. Even with the money, status, and power of this famous and beloved leader, his family had the same struggles as mine. It doesn't matter who you are. In the final analysis, the Reagans are just another loving family trying to deal with the aftermath of AD.

Maureen Reagan has been a particular comfort to me on several occasions. Once on *Good Morning, America*, I could see her pain as she talked lovingly about her father. She even made the comment that those of us who have a family member stricken with AD have a common bond of understanding, and because of it, we are a part of one big family. She also said that we all must support research so that this will be the last generation to suffer the ravages of AD.[6] Even though a medical breakthrough didn't come in time for my mother, there is hope that it will come in time for my generation. I am thankful that God has chosen Maureen Reagan as an instrument to make the public more aware. Her honesty about her situation and her reassuring words have really touched my life.

> The contour of the land
> guides the flow of the river
> while the river carves the land.
> So, we change and are changed by others.
> In this, we are one.

God's Loving Gifts

Sometimes sources of comfort came from unexpected places like the TV set. When I would get really depressed about dealing with Mom's AD and really need God to give me comfort, somehow I would turn on the television at precisely the right moment to hear what I needed to her. I watch *The Oprah Winfrey Show* as often as I can. Toward the end of Mom's illness, the show came on later in our time zone, and I could watch it almost every day when I came home from work. Just the show in general was an anchor to what was happening to everyday people like me all over the United States and the world. All of us have some struggle to endure. With teaching high school English, grading papers at home, cooking, laundry, and grocery shopping, seeing Mom at least once a week in a town forty miles away, along with other things that kept coming up, there was little time left for myself. The "Remembering Your Spirit" portion of the program at the end of the show, if nothing else, reminded me how important it was not to neglect the spiritual part of my being.

I have been retired for a year, and it's hard to imagine how I got all that done. Many women do manage to get all that done and raise children on top of it. Not just women, but men and children are stressed out beyond belief in our modern day struggle to make a living in a two income household while trying to maintain quality family relationships.

Several of Oprah's guests, and Oprah herself, would talk about the importance of learning lessons through the struggles in life. Throughout Mom's progression of AD, I was already beginning to discover on my own that something positive could come out of what I thought was the worst thing I had to experience in my life. In our American culture, we are taught proverbially to "take the bull by the horns" and solve the problem. Problems like a parent's illness and impending death cannot be solved; they have to be endured. Endurance is not only a test of strength and will, but it can be a great catalyst for learning and spiritual growth.

Younger people, by and large, aren't as compassionate as older people because most haven't as yet suffered much loss. Only through our own suffering can we truly have great compassion for others. I think that most teenagers don't truly comprehend their own mortality. This is why statistically teenage drivers are more reckless. When a teen experiences the death of a friend or family member, they too have to face reality about their own eventual death. People shouldn't dwell on suffering and death, but when you realize that you never know what day will be your last, every day becomes a miracle. Most of all, it becomes more urgent to know where you will spend eternity. It somewhat diminishes the importance of what happens in this life in comparison to the hope of what will happen in the next. A seven year struggle with a parent's AD doesn't seem as long when you look back at the experiences they had throughout an entire lifetime. Seven years seem very short indeed when looking toward where you will spend eternity. To me, perspective is so important.

I could see bits of light in the darkness through people I had known for many years, as well as staff members and students at the high school. I retired in May of 2000 after teaching twenty-six years of high school English. Over the years, when I would get discouraged with teaching and try to find some other career, I could never think of anything I thought was more important.

I started teaching in 1973, and I don't think the majority of students have changed in any significant way. Most students and their parents are good and decent people who want to work hard and have a happy life. The big difference is the number of troubled young people. In my early teaching career, I might just have one student in a school year who was considered a big problem. Sometimes I could go a whole year and not have anything major happen. Normal teenagers, as every parent knows, are very challenging to deal with, and problem students can make parenting and teaching even more difficult.

I heard some statistics at a state teachers' convention in the early 1990's, which I will never forget. The speaker said that statistically about five percent of our student population had major problems, but by the year 2000, it would be about twenty percent. That didn't mean that all these students would be troublemakers in class, but it did mean that the teacher would have to deal with them in some special way because of physical, mental, emotional, or spiritual challenges in their lives. As a teacher, of course, I loved to see students do well in their classes, but my best memories revolve around when I could do something to really help a student deal with a difficult problem.

As I got into my fifties, there seemed to be more and more students with bigger and bigger problems. With decreased energy because of my age and dealing with Mom's AD, I started to experience feelings of burnout. Even in a small town like Miami, Oklahoma, staff members knew that we had students who were like powder kegs ready to blow, long before the Columbine-like shootings came to the consciousness of the nation. After the school shootings began to erupt, it was obvious to all that school was no longer a safe place to be. A few students had the attitude that I was just placed there to make their lives miserable and that the homework I assigned was a great interference in their personal lives because of jobs, dates, etc. For some, rules were something to be challenged on a daily basis. I felt sorry for the overwhelming majority of students who had to put up with me dealing with disgruntled students. It took so much time away from learning. I think that the modern schools are especially frustrating for the older teachers who know that there was a better time. I worked under the theory that if teenagers could behave in the past, they could do it now. It paid off eventually, but it took longer and longer as time went by to get the classes organized to have a good learning environment.

One day when all the problems of life seemed to pile up, I looked out into the classroom and saw one or two smiling faces in a sea of sullen faces probably similar to mine. I finally asked one of these students after class why they were so happy when most other people complained and were discontented most of the time. The answer was their spirituality. They loved the Lord and put all their burdens on Him.

Two years before I retired, I had several students invite me to the nationwide event, "See You at the Pole," in which students, not on school time, would gather at the flag pole at their respective schools to pray. A group of students at the First Baptist Church in Miami gathered every Wednesday morning throughout the school year before school to pray around the flag pole when the weather was good or in the main hall when the weather was not. All students were invited to attend. Even though I was getting closer to God all the time, I had not as yet joined a church. I really believe that this is what got me through the last two years of teaching and dealing with my mother's AD. I would hear them say, "Lord, keep us safe" and "Lord, help our teachers" and "Lord, help me to be an example of Christian love to other students who don't know You." Through their prayers, I was reminded of the many good and honest students who struggle to make it in a world not of their own choosing.

Today, students worry about parents' rules, tests, grades, clothes, cars, boyfriends and girlfriends, just like their contemporaries when I first started teaching in 1973. Now, they also have to deal with other students who bring drugs to school, have fights in the hallways in an ever increasing number, and wonder if they too might face a gunman in the halls someday. Their courage and positive attitude gave me strength. They taught me the importance of gathering to pray with other people of faith. I didn't have most of these students in class, and I didn't even know many of their names, but just knowing that there were students and parents out there praying for the good of the school and the community was a great comfort to me. I thank God for this group. It is true that "a child will lead the way."

I also noticed how some of the caring and spiritual staff members at school worked together—sometimes without even knowing it. For example, on the first anniversary of the Oklahoma City bombing, many schools in the state of Oklahoma stopped at the precise time of the bombing (9:02 AM) for a moment of silence. I was very close to a student whose father had just been severely injured in an accident. I didn't know it at the time, but another teacher, who also had a close relationship with this girl, had called another classroom she was in and asked her to come to her room during that moment of silence. The other teacher was afraid that thinking about the bombing, even though the student hadn't known anyone injured or killed, might be upsetting to her on top of all the other emotional upheaval she had been through.

Everyone was to pause at that appointed time for a moment. Something made me look out into the hall, and I saw her standing there frozen. I felt like God led me to the hall to comfort her. We embraced each other without words and stood together for that long, agonizing minute. After the second bell, she said that she was on her way to the other teacher's room in the annex but wasn't able to make it on time before the school-wide announcement. She said that she would be fine and continued on. I called the teacher and told her that the student was on her way. This is just one of the many examples of how God guides people to be at the right place at the right time. I am beginning to believe that there is no such thing as a coincidence.

One of my greatest gifts is my husband Arley. My first husband Rob died in 1987 at the age of forty-two of a massive heart attack. As time passed after Rob's death, I hoped that I would find someone to help me through my mother's aging, decline, and death. I knew that I couldn't do it alone. I have no biological children, and I knew it would only be a matter of time because of her advanced age. It wasn't exactly a prayer but a strong thought in my mind. The Lord gave me exactly the husband I needed anyway. Arley and I were married less than a year after we met. I didn't know much about him as I should have. I kept thinking that I should check into his background, and later he said that he had the same thoughts. We were so busy having fun and making plans that we never got around to it. After I met his friends and family and he met mine, we both knew that we could trust each other. He always prayed at supper time, which I hadn't done on a regular basis for many years.

The one thing that impressed me most about him was that he had taken care of his mother Ruth for over forty years. His father remarried and then died at the age of fifty-four. Since he was the oldest child, his father asked him to look after her. She started showing signs of a mental condition when Arley was in early adolescence and had to be hospitalized on several occasions. It was back in the days before medication could allow someone like her to lead somewhat of a normal life in the community. As she got older, she was cared for in nursing homes. Arley was always there to visit as often as he could and take care of her needs. It occurred to me that anyone like him who was so devoted to taking care of his mother had to be a good person. I was right.

After several years passed and my Mom started showing signs of AD, he was a great help in supporting me. When I first took her to Medicalodge, I told him one day that I didn't know if I could take it anymore. Of course, I knew that I would never desert her. He told me that my job would be done only when she was in her grave and not before. I started thinking about all the years that he had looked after his mother, and I knew that with his help and with God's help, I could endure it.

Being married to Arley brought another surprise. Arley has two grown sons, Randy and Mike, who have brought another joyful dimension to my life. Since I never had any children of my own, naturally the prospect of having a grandchild never entered my consciousness. Mike's son Jeremiah has truly been an unexpected gift. When he was younger, Mom and he were very close.

The last year before Mom died, I told him that she was really losing ground mentally. I said, "Remember when you two used to be good friends?" He answered, "We still are." Isn't it wonderful that God sometimes gives us even more than we ever expected to have or know that we needed?

A Place of Refuge and Hope

As the years went by and Mom continued her slow decline, I started thinking about what would happen after her death. Most people are familiar with the Precious Moments figurines of the cute, innocent children with the big eyes created by the very talented artist Sam Butcher. The national headquarters for Precious Moments was built in Carthage, Missouri, which is about forty miles from my home. When people would come to visit from out of state, I would take them on a tour. I went there so many times over the years that when I was in despair dealing with my Mom's AD, it eventually became a place of refuge and comfort for me.

Besides gift shops and a restaurant, the main attraction is the Precious Moments chapel. Mr. Butcher painted angels, which resemble the wide-eyed children in the figurines, on the high ceiling of the chapel. He lay on his back for many hours to complete his work on scaffolding like Michelangelo did when he painted the famous Sistine Chapel. The Precious Moments children appear in all forms of art in the chapel and in areas such as the brass tablets on both sides of the front entrance that depict scenes from the Old and the New Testament, carvings on the wooden chapel doors, and a colorful array of stained glass windows.

On the very large front wall of the chapel, Mr. Butcher painted a variety of Precious Moments figures residing in his whimsical version of heaven, which he calls Hallelujah Square. The Precious Moments figure inside the gate to heaven, who must have been new on the job, holds a sign upside down which reads, "Welcome." Another one holds a heart that has been taped back together. It is an inspiring depiction of how we will be made whole when we enter heaven. The guide always tells the story of how the only figure that is life-like is Christ. When Mr. Butcher painted Christ, he unknowingly painted Jesus in the exact center of the huge wall in the front of the chapel. He believes that this happened because Christ should be the center of our lives.

In my mind I could see my mother as a Precious Moments figure with gray hair holding a book with the words "Memory Book" on the front because I knew her memory would be restored in heaven. This image in my mind gave me great comfort every time I went. It helped me picture a time when she, as well as all the rest of us, will be happy, peaceful, and joined with our loved ones. We will at last "have a Precious Moment with the Lord in Hallelujah Square." His painting, in turn, inspired me to write this poem:

Hallelujah Square

> No more tears
> No more sorrow
> No more fears
> About tomorrow.
> No rent to pay
> No bills to meet
> Jump on a cloud
> And tap your feet.
> When we all meet someday
> In Hallelujah Square.
>
> We won't need canes.
> The lame will walk.

Praise the Lord.
The mute will talk.
Illness gone
With pain unheard.
The deaf will hear
God's Holy Word
When we all meet someday
In Hallelujah Square.

Walk on down
Life's bumpy road.
Touch a heart.
Lift a load.
Spread love around
To all you see.
A place awaits
And I'll see you there
For a Precious Moment with the Lord
In Hallelujah Square.

      Judith Ames David

Special Moments

With the long and often agonizing progression of AD, it seems that I continued to grieve each new stage. Just as I got used to the mild short term memory loss, the progression of Mom's disease would accelerate to a new level. I was somewhat comforted by the fact that at least she still knew who I was. In the later stages of AD, sometimes I was me; sometimes I was her sister. As her memory loss became more pronounced, she remembered more what I looked like around ten years before with dark brown or salt and pepper hair. Now I was almost gray. I was beginning to look more like the older members of our family—most of whom had departed this earth many years ago. Then I figured I didn't care who she thought I was, as long as it was someone she loved.

During the last two years or so, of course, she didn't know me most of the time. Many times I would think that she hugged me in a special way, and then I would notice that she hugged the staff members in much the same way. It hurt; on the other hand, I was glad that when I wasn't around, she had other people there she cared for and who cared for her. This was a real lesson in unconditional love—to love her and not be sure if she knew to love me back. I knew she couldn't help it, and in her right state of mind, she would have. One time she looked at me and called me Mom. She looked at me with so much love in her big blue eyes because she hadn't seen her mother for so long since her mom had died when I was in grade school. I remember her crying a few days after the funeral while she was sweeping up after taking down our Christmas tree so many years ago. Because I was a young child, she looked at me and quit crying. This helped me know that even though she was very sad about her mother, she had to go on for the rest of us—just as I would be forced to go on without her some day.

Much of the knowledge I gained about AD and was motivated to keep learning was in response to what my mother had been and was experiencing. I learned that no one actually dies of AD but from the complications such as infection, pneumonia, dehydration, malnutrition, or other conditions that slowly shut down major systems in the body. Of course, the brain controls all physical function, and so AD affects everything. Her ability to walk was a blessing and a curse. She exhibited a phenomena known as sundowners. Some AD patients become more confused and agitated when the sun goes down. It is even harder to process reality with the lower light levels at night, and the fact that most elderly people have failing eyesight really compounds the problem. Like very young children, sometimes they just get their days and nights mixed up. She would often wander up and down the halls until past midnight. No one could stop her. No one at Medicalodge tried to stop her. It was their policy to give the residents as much freedom as possible and to be flexible about the residents' sometimes irregular sleeping patterns.

She had also lost her appetite. Sometimes, AD patients fail to recognize they are hungry or simply lose interest in eating. The increasing need to wander, along with the decreasing appetite, caused her to be in a never ending battle to keep a normal weight. In addition, she was now ninety, and her age was simply catching up with her.

In November of 1999, Mom went into the hospital in Neosho, Missouri, because of an infection, which resulted in dehydration. She was unresponsive when I took her to Emergency that night. Although she remained that way throughout the night and the following morning, they brought her lunch the next day. I looked at it wishing she could eat it when I noticed movement out of the corner of my eye. Her arms shot out for a hug, and she whispered, "You're a wonderful child." She hadn't known me for so long. I know that this was a special gift from God.

During an interview on *Good Morning America*, Maureen Reagan said that when she visited her father, she always wore her red fingernail polish because the former president liked the bright colors so much. She thought that this was one sign that he recognized who she was.[7] We all hang onto that bit of recognition.

During the last year, it became harder and harder for her to finish a sentence, but whenever a child would come around, she came alive. My husband's mother Ruth was in the same nursing home, and she liked listening to gospel singers when they came to visit the facility. Arley's father had been a Pentecostal minister, and she and her sisters had sung in church when she was younger. Eventually, Arley and I learned to live in the past with both of them.

In March of 2000 around three months before she died, it was a warm spring day and a perfect time for a ride around town. Neosho, Missouri, is a beautiful little town, especially in the spring and fall. In the glow of the warming sun, redbud trees and pink and white dogwoods dot the hillsides. Yellow forsythia compete with the yellow of the daffodils. Tulips bloom in colors bright as a kindergarten classroom. The grass is as green as an Irish shamrock. After leaving Big Springs Park, which is only blocks to the old town square with the court house in the center, and listening to the whoosh of the rushing water of a small waterfall gushing from the springs, it was time for a double hot fudge sundae. I put in her favorite music tape, the Mills Brothers. With one hand on the steering wheel and the other holding hers, we sang "Up the Lazy River" to the top of our lungs. We sang,

"Blue skies up above, everyone's in love. Up the lazy river with me." When the tape clicked off, she looked at me and said in a voice as sweet as an angel, "I like being with you." Even though I don't think she knew who I was, I knew she liked my company. I figured that she just chose to love me all over again.

When language goes, hugs become more important. Sometimes, I knew what Mom wanted because I knew her, and sometimes I just had to guess by the look on her face. The language of the spirit is seldom logical and not always spoken.

Nursing Home Angels

*L*ooking for an appropriate nursing home for an active Alzheimer's patient like my mother was a real challenge. Caring for an elderly person's physical health is something that nursing homes were created to do. As the average life expectancy has continued to increase over the years, more and more people and family members have to deal with the decision of how to care for their elderly loved ones when they are no longer able to care for themselves. Some nursing homes let AD patients be in the same area as other patients. Ankle bracelets or some other alerting device sets off an alarm if the resident tries to walk out the door, but my mother was simply too physically active. It would have been a full time job just to keep her safe inside. AD patients in beds or wheelchairs do not have to be in a special section because of their physical limitations.

I visited several AD units in towns surrounding Miami. One was just a wing of an existing nursing home. Another locked unit had a courtyard area at the end of a long hallway, which was really nice, but I didn't see any patients in it, even though the weather was beautiful that day. The nurse on duty said, "I really like to work on this wing because it is so quiet." I thought to myself, "It wouldn't be very quiet if Mom were here." Then I started to realize why it was so quiet. Everyone was just sitting in their chairs not saying a word, even when the nurse tried to get them to speak. I felt like several of them were over-medicated. Many AD patients quit talking, but it seemed a little odd that almost no one was moving around or making noise of any kind. I later learned that medication is crucial in controlling moods to give the AD patients as much quality of life as possible. The doctor and the nursing home staff have to do a real balancing act—not too much and not too little. Too much medication makes some patients as inactive as zombies while too little medication makes others distraught and/ or uncontrollable.

Arley's mother Ruth was already a resident of Medicalodge in Neosho, Missouri. Because he worked in the Neosho area, it was convenient for him to stop by and see her on his way home. It was a forty minute drive from Miami, and I wanted Mom closer to me. When I couldn't find any place acceptable, I finally considered the AD unit at Medicalodge. It was a large wing with two halls perpendicular to one another with the nurses' station at the right angle in the middle. Although the unit was locked for safety reasons, a patient could walk down either long hall into a very large courtyard with flowers, bird feeders, benches, and a gazebo. Many of the healthier AD patients wandered around a great deal, and so the courtyard gave them a very beautiful, stimulating but relaxing place to go when the weather permitted. Also, with the short term memory loss, they really didn't get bored walking back and forth over the same area. At least, it gave them an illusion of freedom.

The atmosphere at Medicalodge was very different from the other nursing homes I had visited. Many residents were sitting quietly like in the other facilities, but others were talking and moving about at will. It was louder and somewhat chaotic in comparison, but the point is that they were doing what they wanted to do within reason. This is a great deal more work for the staff, but the residents were allowed to be themselves. This is not an easy philosophy. The staff must care for people who have the mental capacity of toddlers and grade school children while giving them the respect of an adult. These grown up toddlers are also frail with tenuous balance and bones that are more easily broken. Like children, they would get frustrated and throw tantrums. When they did, the staff members would skillfully redirect them. They would use medication to calm them only when absolutely necessary and other methods had been exhausted.

After Dad's death in the early 70's, my mother had lived on her own for many years. At first it was difficult, if not impossible, for her to understand why someone was telling her what to do. In addition, most residents in AD units don't remember where they are or why they are there. If I had a dollar for every time I heard, "I want to go home," I wouldn't be rich, but I could afford longer or more luxurious vacations. They don't see anyone familiar and often feel deserted no matter how many times they are told that their family members are only a phone call away. Staff members have to answer the same questions over and over from many different residents. Working at a nursing home in general, and at an AD unit in particular, is a real calling from God. I can find no other explanation for this unlimited patience on the part of the staff.

At the end of my career, I had taught high school for twenty-six years, but nothing prepared me for this kind of fortitude. High school students are very trying at times, but I knew that someday they would grow out of it and become responsible adults like most of the rest of us. I could remember how unfinished I was at that age. To me, this was a different reality. As time passed, there would be only decline. I'm just glad that God made all different kinds of people so that we would all like different kinds of jobs. At this unit, no one restricted the patients unless it was a danger to them or to another resident or staff member. The staff members were attentive to the residents' needs, talked to them, and in general showed them a great deal of affection and respect.

Although nurses are professionals, they never get the money they deserve. Most nursing home workers of all kinds could make almost as much money working at Wal-Mart and get better benefits. So what was the difference? I found out later that all the people who worked in the unit had special training in how to deal with patients who suffered from AD and other dementia, and most of the staff chose to be on that wing.

When I was a new teacher, I was under the mistaken belief that I could do a good job and that the high school would run smoothly as long as all the teachers were dedicated to their jobs. I was fortunate to have one of my best principals for my first principal. He probably made it look too easy. When I got into situations where leadership was lacking, it was only then that I realized that a good leader really does set the tone for the rest of the staff. Apparently, this is also true of nursing homes.

Evelyn Hottinger, the nursing home administrator, held this belief. "You don't have to be a Christian to work here, but you must have a Christian attitude." She set an example by working hard and not tolerating anyone who didn't. Working hard was not enough, though, because staff members were expected to treat each patient in the AD unit and the skilled nursing wing with respect and affection, which was not always easy to do.

A competent caring staff is hard to find. You can't fake that. Of course, staff members tend to be a little friendlier and more caring when family members are around. At times I would walk in quietly when no one knew I was on the premises. I would almost always without exception hear kind words and sense a caring attitude. I often witnessed my mother's reaction towards the people who worked there, and it was always positive. If she had been uncomfortable living there, believe me everyone would have known it. They worked very hard to help the residents feel like they were home. Evelyn was always willing to work with people to help them do a better job, but she did not tolerate anyone who cared more about their own problems than the well being of the residents.

The people who worked directly with the residents had the proverbial patience of Job. The activities department often kept my mother-in-law Ruth busy in the common area just outside the AD unit because she liked to do crafts, go to the nursing home church activities, and sing gospel music. Mom couldn't participate in many activities because her attention span was short, and besides she was so physically active that she would simply walk away. She was still given a great deal of attention. She would get snacks whenever she was hungry. Even laundry workers would stop and chat with her, and housekeeping would let her watch them work at night when she couldn't sleep. Sometimes she liked to push around the trash barrels on rollers in the hall. At times she might push them into closets, and housekeeping couldn't find them. They just laughed and commented on what a character she was. This kept her occupied at night when all the other residents were in bed. She eventually would give up and go to bed. It was her home, and she could live as she pleased.

I really admire the family members who can care for their loved one in their homes, but not everyone can. When I would feel guilty about not being able to care for her in our home, Arley would remind me that it took three shifts of professionally trained people to care for her and others like her. I always was and forever will be grateful to every one of these nursing home angels.

A Bit of Humor

When I was a teenager, I was often suspicious that some of my friends came to my house to visit my mother as much to visit with me. I didn't know whether to take this as a compliment or not. Several of my friends even called her Mom. Mom was like the character Estelle Getty played on the TV show, *The Golden Girls,* and I have always been the more serious daughter. She talked me into bleaching my hair in my junior year of high school because she never got to do it when she was young. When someone would ask her what she thought about the changes in music or fashion, she would just say, "Well, you gotta keep up with the times."

If anyone would criticize young people for kiddish pranks, she would tell about the time her cousins brought a pony into the house. My favorite story is about her escapade with a camera when she was a young child. According to her, she ran all over the neighborhood taking pictures of people, knowing there was no film in the camera. Back in those days, getting your picture taken was more of an occasion, and most people were lucky to own a camera. Mothers cleaned up and dressed up their children in anticipation of a lasting image for future generations. Several weeks later her mother was plagued by questions about when the film would be developed and the pictures would be ready. My grandmother was then left with the embarrassing job of telling everyone that there had been no film in the camera. Mom wasn't proud of her photographic adventure that bewildered other people. She just wanted to remind parents of today that we were not perfect as children either. Although she was an intelligent and responsible woman, she always retained her childlike curiosity and wonder. If anyone was young at heart, my mother was.

I would never make fun of anything my mother or anyone else said or did who was suffering from AD or other dementia, but I do believe that within limits you have to see humor in some situations to keep yourself from going insane. Sometimes, one has to laugh to keep from crying. Anyway, Mom always liked a good laugh, even if it was at her own expense, as long as people did it in a loving way.

I noticed that Mom eventually lost all concept of how old she was, especially the last two years before her death. In the morning when she had a great deal more energy, I would ask her how old she was. One time she said she was fifty-five. I said, "That's funny because I'm your daughter, and I'm fifty-three. By the end of the day when she was tired, she usually reported to be in her seventies. She, of course, was in her eighties. Physically, she really never felt as old as she really was.

It's hard to pin down when the short term memory loss eroded into the long term memory. One day I caught her looking very puzzled into the mirror. I asked her what was wrong. Probably noticing her many wrinkles, she said, "I have to do something about my face."

Mom was always a very kind and loving person, but she did have an ornery side. She had always been known to mutter comments under her breath. As she progressed more and more into AD, she no longer censored many of her comments, and with her slight hearing loss, some comments were loud enough to be heard. Once while walking down the hall, she passed by one of the residents and said, "She sure has a big butt!" Before she got adjusted to living in the

AD wing of the nursing home, she would look at the aides and nurses and say, "Who do they think they are?" I would just say, "They're the people who take care of you, Mom."

Along with the short term memory loss, Mom's eyesight started to dim even more because of cataracts. It's hard to figure out the world when afflicted with AD, and the loss of vision doesn't help any. One day at the nursing home, we were sitting in the dining area getting ready to eat lunch. She must have been remembering back to a time when she had to feed a crowd of people at her home and said, "Is there enough to eat for everyone? Had we better go to the grocery store?" Of course, I assured her that there was enough for all.

Medicalodge has a small dining area in the AD unit that could pass for a section in a regular restaurant. At first Mom wondered where to pay for the meal. I have heard several residents over the years expressing concern over paying for what they received. I usually told Mom that it was a very nice place to eat, and we would just put it on our bill and pay it at the end of the month, which, in essence, was true.

In March of 2000, only about five months before she passed away, one of the nurses asked if I would like to see some pictures of Margaret. They had them taped on the other side of the counter at the nurses' station. One was of her in a bright orange Starter jacket. I said that it was a cute picture and nice of the owner of the jacket to put it on her. Apparently, she had just seen it on a rack and proudly put it on. "Go, Mama!" The other two pictures were of Mom pushing another resident around in a wheel chair. She was ninety herself at the time. She would often go to the nurses' station to report that some other resident needed help. She apparently still liked to help other people, even if the other person didn't know they needed it. I was so glad the staff had a sense of humor too. I don't see how you could survive working in an AD unit without one.

This story should be under the heading of: "Sometimes

things aren't as bad as they seem." I looked back at the first day I took Mom to the nursing home as one of the hardest and worst days of my life. Arley and I had brought her clothes into her room, but I had to leave for a short while because it was all I could do to keep from crying right in front of her. I wanted her to adjust to the new place, and I wasn't sure if she would understand why I was crying. I just knew it would not help the situation. I hugged her and then took off to the car for a good sob. After Mom had been in the nursing home for over three years and about two weeks before her death, I talked to Millie, one of the CNA's, about the day I brought her in.

I said, "That was quite a day."

She replied, "That was quite a day for all of us."

"I was really upset, and I'm sure she was really upset after I left."

"I don't know if she was upset or not, but she did set off the fire alarm."

"Oh, my, she felt so bad she resorted to that."

Millie couldn't suppress a chuckle. "Felt bad? She was hiding behind a corner laughing. It was hard to explain to the police and fire department what had happened."

For a while after I found out, we all called her "Four Alarm Margaret." I remembered back over the years how many times before her illness she had kidded about setting off a fire alarm, but, of course, her rational mind stopped her. Nothing stopped her this time.

Nursing home staff members have a special calling, especially the ones who work in an AD unit. It's like having toddlers wandering all over the place, often asking the same questions over and over again. However, these are toddlers you have to treat with respect. It's a tough job, and it takes the patience of an earthly angel to do it with grace, love, and a bit of humor.

Lines from the All School Play

Adrenaline alerts my legs and brain.
I rush back to school.
Forgot the combination to the locker
I can't find in the blur of sameness.
The door slams itself behind me.
There is no way out.
The lines from the all school play
melt from memory.
I'm the mechanical ballerina
on my mother's music box,
dizzy from performing.
My ankles collapse in upon themselves.
In the dark, I reach for a doorknob
that isn't there.
A mad man chases the shadow that is me
through long resonating corridors
that convulse right and left without end.
I hold tightly to a pillar made of smoke.
The sweet smell of incense
invades the cool layer of mist
that stuns my momentum,
but the spider cheers me on.
With clutching kindness
it devours me without thought.

                                      Judith Ames David

Lines from the All School Play

I wrote this poem around fifteen years ago before Christ came into my life in real and personal way. Some might call this defining experience "walking with the Lord," "feeling God's presence," or even "being saved." Before writing this poem, I had read a book about tapping into the right side of the brain to release subconscious thoughts. It is what educators and others call brainstorming. In one exercise I was to come up with a word and then write down thoughts as quickly as I could without being censored by the more logical left side of the brain. Then I was to somehow (they didn't say how) switch over to the left side of the brain to actually write the poem. At this time I could delete, add to, and polish.

This clustering method can be used to discover new and fresh ways of saying things, or it may perhaps tell you something about yourself you may not have known. Anyway, from a long list of thoughts about fear, I constructed this seemingly nonsensical poem I titled, "Lines from the All School Play," because one of the recurring dreams I have had most of my life was being in a play and experiencing the embarrassment of forgetting my lines in front of an audience full of people.

I decided to put my fears into a school setting since I have either attended school or taught school most of my life. Over the years I have discovered different interpretations of what this poem might mean to my conscious mind. Several things were obvious to me right away. The second stanza talks about "the blur of sameness" of conformity that tends to lock up or hide us from our real selves. More recently, I have interpreted it to mean that I was lost in my conformity to the ways of the world. My ankles collapsing in upon themselves like something sinking into a black hole in space was about my fear of public speaking in high school, college, and beyond. I could make myself not look afraid, but I could hardly maintain my balance to stand and give a speech because my ankles would get weak from stage fright.

As I got closer to God, I started to understand how this poem relates to my spirituality. I now believe that the shadow chased by a mad man represents the dark side of my nature, the unforgiven. I am now convinced that the "loud, resonating corridors that convulse right and left without end" show that I am in the belly of the beast. Originally, I thought that the pillar of smoke represented my trying to hold onto things without substance. Now, I feel that it has a double meaning, then unknown to me. As God lead Moses and the Israelites out of bondage, He went ahead of them and guided them with a pillar of cloud by day and a pillar of fire by night. Both pillars guided them by day and by night because it was the real presence of our God who will never desert us in troubled times.

The smell of incense in my poem, I believe, is another indication of God's presence. In Exodus 40 God instructs Moses in setting up the Tabernacle, and Moses places the gold altar of incense in the Tabernacle. Also, in Psalm 141:2, David says: "My prayer be set before you like incense..."

I now think that the spider that "cheered me on" represented all my fears that kept me in a constant state of agitation, keeping my spirit dead and away from Christ. After all, fear is the opposite of faith. The "clutching kindness" reminds me of the grasp of the great deceiver. The end of the poem is frightening to me because I was consumed by my fear when I had already been devoured by the beast. This is just a taste of what Hell would be like where the torture is ever present for eternity. Spiritually, because of the lack of Christ in my life, I was sure to repeat the same scenario described in this poem over and over again. The good news is that even when I was lost in the belly of the beast and dead in spirit, the Lord's love and guidance was still immediately available to me if only I had reached out to receive it.

Wrestling with Guilt

*I*n my case, wrestling with guilt seems to be a more accurate description of what I did and still continue to do. Even now, over eight months since my mother passed away, I wonder if I could have said more or done more. Ironically, she died the summer after I retired. I finally would have had more time to spend with her. I could have brought her home more often. There are times when I would give anything to have just one more day with her. My guilty feelings, from what I have heard and read about, are somewhat normal in the grieving process, as long as they are not all-consuming. The feelings still remain, but to a lesser degree as time goes on. All I can do is continue to pray for that "peace that passeth all understanding."

After Mom started living at Medicalodge, I was in the middle of a storm of guilt that rumbled and flashed through my mind in waves of constant agitation. About a year after she started living there, I attended the usual teachers' workshops in August, a few days before the start of the school year. They hired a speaker, whose name I don't remember, probably on purpose. Over the years I have been motivated by many educational speakers. It did always help to get me "back in the groove" of dealing with a hundred or more teenagers a day. This time was different.

Mostly, the main speaker just spouted platitudes about what is wrong with America, after which the audience would clap in agreement. After all these years in education, I felt that it is always easier to point out what is wrong than it is to offer solutions and work to try to put them into practice. I listened anyway. His voice boomed out into the auditorium, "What is wrong with a country that puts its elderly in nursing homes instead of taking care of them at home?" The audience applauded wildly. I was one of the older teachers, and I was sure that most educators there had not had to deal with an aging parent and didn't know what was involved. I was in my early fifties and dealing with it much younger than some, and I was still working. My first thoughts were that no one should criticize me or anyone else in the same situation until they had proverbially "walked a mile in my shoes."

I really admire people who do stay home and take care of the elderly. It was just not my choice to quit work. Even if I had quit work, taking care of an active AD patient is something that would have been twenty-four/seven. She could have wandered off at any time. It would have entailed my watching her day and night. Now in retrospect, I know that I would have had to deal with this situation for an extended period of time because of the slow progression of this disease in my mother's case. Anyway, this is a decision that family members have to make, and I don't think others should criticize unless they know what it is like. Family members experience enough heartache already. Saying this, I didn't intend to just dump her off at a nursing home. Even if I couldn't take care of her at home, my family and I were committed to visiting her as often as we could and taking care of her needs.

On one end of the scale, there is the family member who devotes his or her entire life taking care of the AD patient, and on the other end of the scale are family members who seldom, if ever, visit their loved ones. I don't know why people abandon their parents or family members. Maybe their relationship wasn't as close as ours was with our mother. I know there are many other obligations in life. I think one of the reasons people avoid nursing homes is because they hate to see their family member in that condition. It is very painful, and it also reminds us of our own aging and death.

I earned an MS degree in high school counseling and have always loved reading psychology and self-help books. I easily understood the psychological defense mechanisms like rationalization (making excuses) and projection (blaming the tennis racket for a bad game), but I always had trouble understanding the concept of approach/avoidance. Somehow, it just never did make much sense to me until Mom started her decline into AD. When I visited her, at times I wanted to be home because of how sad it made me feel. When I was at home, I wanted to be there with her. I never felt like I was doing enough no matter what.

A few things helped. My teaching experience helped give me patience in communicating with students with a great variety of language abilities. As Mom's ability to communicate declined, this skill was very useful. My counseling degree helped me to understand my guilt, real or imagined, and the anticipatory grief I was feeling because of her decline and eventual death. Nothing, however, totally took away the pain of loss and guilt. I found solace wherever I could.

I found comfort in talking to other people who were in a similar situation. Knowing that I wasn't alone in my struggle really helped. Evelyn, the nursing home administrator, also reminded me that Mom had already experienced her prime years, and that Arley and I shouldn't miss out on ours. She said that she had seen grown children get tied down to looking after their parents for so many years that they never had quality time in their lives to enjoy the freedom of their own retirement. Some of these older children could be in their sixties and seventies and become very ill shortly after the parent died. She was not suggesting that we not spend time with our mothers. She was just reminding us that life really is a balancing act at times.

God's timing is perfect, isn't it? It seems that people

come back into my life at precisely the right time. I first met Joan Isom around fifteen years ago when she was part of the Oklahoma State Arts Council's Artist-In-Residence program. She facilitated a poetry and creative writing workshop at Jay, Oklahoma, where I taught high school English at the time. She also encouraged me when I first started writing poetry. She would offer many suggestions, and I'm glad that I had the sense to listen. Listening to constructive criticism from someone who knows what they're talking about is the only way a beginner can improve.

In December of 1999, she invited us to a Christmas open house. I was so disappointed I couldn't make it because I was ill. I was anxious to talk to her about a book that she and Mary Anne Maier had co-edited called, *The Leap Years: Women Reflect on Change, Loss, and Love*. This book came into my awareness right when I needed it the most. Even though I couldn't go to the open house, I bought and read the book as soon as I could get to a bookstore. Through these essays, I saw myself struggling with many of the same issues because I was in the transitional period between adulthood and old age and also due to the life circumstances dealing with my mother's extended illness.

One essay in particular helped me to put my guilt into perspective. The following is taken from *The Crosswicks Journal: Book Two* entitled *The Summer of the Great-Grandmother*, in which the award winning author Madeleine L'Engle examines her false guilt concerning her own mother's decline. The excerpt is from a chapter entitled, "Ouisa: The Realness of Things." After talking with a humanist friend, the author believes, unlike her friend, that since God is in control, she no longer has to experience a false guilt concerning something over which she has no control. As most people, I recognize that we have control over many things in our lives. Remember the old adage: "God helps those who help themselves." On the other hand, we must recognize the areas in which we have no control, and I believe that my first step in becoming a more mature Christian was giving that control over to God. Like most people, I find myself trying to take back that control and then quickly realizing that the reason I gave it to God in the first place was because I couldn't do it on my own.

In the following excerpt, she contrasts her belief in God, who she believes is in control of the universe, with a humanist friend who believes that she is totally in control of her destiny.

> It is a trap we all fall into on occasion, but it is particularly open to the intelligent atheist. There is no God and if there is, he's not arranging things very well; therefore, I must be in charge. If I don't succeed, if I am not perfect, I carry the weight of the whole universe on my shoulders.[8]

Through her most wise words, I learned to hand even my feelings of false guilt over to the Lord. These negative feelings are so destructive. At a time like that, I realized that it was important for me to try to maintain a balanced life for my own sake and for my mother's sake. For one thing, she loved me and would not want to be the reason for my spiritual, psychological, or physical downfall. For another, if the family members burn out, they are of no use to the AD patient.

Doris, a lifelong friend of Arley's family who lives in Odessa, Texas, recently e-mailed us celebrating her last radiation treatment for cancer. In it, she refers to Isaiah 40:29–31. She says: "And we can make it through the storms if we rise above the storm and let it carry us on strong wings like the eagles. I love you and hope that you have the empowerment to see you through the storms that may come your way." Her words were a great reminder to me that only God can help us rise above the storms in our lives.

He gives strength to the weary
and increases the power of the weak.
Even youths grow tired and weary,
and young men stumble and fall;
but those who hope in the Lord
will renew their strength.
They will soar on wings like eagles,
they will run and not grow weary,
they will walk and not be faint.

                                      Isaiah 40:29–31

Spiritual Growth

Why me? During the time of any life changing event, most people ponder this question. I was no exception. All throughout the seven years, I tried to understand why this was happening to her and the rest of the family. When she was dying, people would say, "She's ninety-one. She's lived a very long life." I was grateful for that. Since she was an older mother, thirty-seven when I was born, I was blessed to have her for so long. My mind could comprehend this, but my heart said, "My mother is not a statistic, and she certainly has never been old to me." One thing I knew for sure was that all people must die, but this was not the way I wanted my mother to spend her last years. We all pray for a quick and dignified death since it must come. As time went by, I started to think about what I was learning from this major life experience. Then I thought of all the people in the Bible whose faith was tested. Job was tested over and over and remained faithful. I was not better than he, was I? I was no longer angry at God. The reverse was true. I was beginning to depend on Him more and more every day. My mother's illness started to make some sense, at least in my mind.

During this time, I really learned the meaning of unconditional love. Toward the end when Mom didn't know who I was, it seemed like I was just visiting her body. Sometimes I wondered why I even bothered to go see her when she didn't know me from anyone else. I was never sorry I did. There was always something I could do for her or for someone else like her. The help in all nursing homes changes fairly often. When you couple this with memory loss, most residents are unable to fully comprehend who works there and who are only visitors. Often a resident would ask for water or would seek attention in some other way. I would help whoever needed it, and I noticed other family members would do the same. It was comforting to know that when I wasn't there, many other people would show my mother kindness.

One day a lady lying in bed saw me in the hall and asked, "Would you pull the blanket over me? I'm cold." I remember how I liked to be tucked in bed as a child. I made an extra special fuss over her, kissed her, and said, "Good night, Ruby. I love you." Before my mother had the same illness, I might have just walked by and told the aides because it wasn't my job or because I needed to tend to my mother and get on my way. Now, I really understood what Maureen Reagan had said. We truly are all part of one big family because of our common experience. I think it is true of most people who go through any trying experience whether it be AD, a terminal illness, or the death of a loved one. Only when we suffer, do we feel more compassion for others.

What I thought was the worst thing that could possibly happen to me in my life turned out to be the most life-changing. Mom has always loved children. She was disappointed as a young woman when her doctor told her that she wouldn't be able to have any. When she did, she treated us as her treasures. As a child, I did what she said most of the time, not because I was afraid of her but because I didn't want to disappoint her. I was not the perfect teenager, and I didn't tell her everything I did, but somehow her unconditional love kept me from crossing too far over the line. At any time during her life, I think that if God had asked her if she would suffer for her children's sake, she would not have hesitated and would have answered a resounding "yes." I'm not saying that her AD was just for my sake, but I am saying that because of our mutual struggle, I became closer to God. In my mind anyway, my having to watch her seven years of decline at least made some sense. It affected other family members in different ways, but all I can tell you about is what it did to me and for me.

As the years went on, I started to depend more and more on God's love and guidance. I could not have made it through without prayer and relying on His awesome power and strength. Without this strength, I think I would have either lost my physical health or emotional well-being. What at first seemed to be a disaster later on turned out to be the greatest gift—the gift of salvation.

I know that I look at her through the eyes of a daughter, but everyone who met her liked her right away. Although she was intelligent, she wasn't the smartest person in the world. She was very cute standing five feet two inches with blue eyes that sparkled with mischief, and her head was crowned with shimmering white hair. But she was not physically the most beautiful person I had seen. She certainly wasn't rich or powerful. So what was the attraction? I believe that it was her honesty, her love for people, her love of life, and a great love for God that radiated from her face.

From this point of view, I was able to somewhat remove myself from the pain of witnessing the last part of her life and how it had caused anguish to me and the rest of my family. I continued to learn and grow throughout this ordeal. At times I was so busy figuratively falling down the stairs that I couldn't figure out how to keep from falling down the stairs. Not being close to God is emotionally exhausting. I know I couldn't have made it on my own. My growing faith in the Lord was the glue that held me together during this trying time. I don't think that everyone has to suffer to be brought to the Lord, but sometimes suffering—whether it be physical, emotional, or spiritual—does just that. In Romans 5:1–4, we see a purpose in suffering when we turn to the Lord for help and hope.

> Therefore since we have been justified through faith, we have peace with God through our Lord Jesus Christ through whom we have gained access by faith into his grace in which we now stand. And we rejoice in our sufferings, because we know that suffering produces perseverance; perseverance, character; and character, hope.

After Mom's death I joined Elk River Baptist Church in Grove, Oklahoma, where we plan to retire and enrolled in a Bible study class called, "The Vision of His Glory." In this study, with the aid of a video and a workbook entitled *The Vision of His Glory: Finding Hope Through the Revelation of Jesus Christ*, Anne Graham Lotz, the daughter of Billy Graham, examines the book of Revelation. Being a former English teacher, I was eager to analyze the vast symbolism. She did discuss some of the symbolic meaning in Revelation, but her main focus was as the title suggested, "A Vision of His Glory." She said that in the busyness of life, we can all lose touch with God. As a new church member, I knew that I would forget to pray on a daily basis and in comparison to her and many other people, I was just a baby spiritually. I was somewhat surprised that the daughter of Billy Graham would say that she had gone through a period of time when she wasn't as close to God as she felt she should have been. After thinking that, I realized that we are all very human and must struggle every day of our lives to remain spiritually fit.

Apparently, she had experienced a string of life-changing events in her immediate family, along with her already busy schedule with church work of various kinds. She made the point that even when we spend a great deal of time in church and doing good for others, we can still lose that personal relationship with Christ. When John was imprisoned on the island of Patmos, his life changed in a dramatic way. He was old, removed from his ministry, and isolated from everything and everyone he loved. She pointed out that if John had not been imprisoned on the island of Patmos and forced to be alone with his thoughts, he would not have received his vision of Christ's glory.[9]

Just like John, major life circumstances stop us and make us look at our lives in a different way. Without my mother's AD, I don't think I would have cried out to the Lord for help. Many times we don't understand why we have to suffer physically, emotionally, or spiritually, but if we are honest about our feelings and face life realistically, we find ourselves changed and stronger at the end. I know that I was brought to a new level of understanding and awareness and a deeper spirituality. Although we as humans will never truly comprehend the power and glory of God, we can learn to depend on Him for our salvation and strength to endure the many trying times in our lives.

A Season to Remember

Although we were unaware of it at the time, Christmas of 1999 was to be the last holiday season we would all spend with Mom. My brother Carlos and his daughter Carla came to our farm for a holiday visit. The brightly colored packages were unwrapped in the glow of the Christmas tree, and I performed my annual burning of the marshmallows on top of the candied yams. After dinner we were so full we could hardly walk, but we all made it into the living room to rest and digest.

Carla sat close to her grandma with one arm around her as she flipped through a book I had on the coffee table. I had bought it in the closing days of 1999 because it briefly described the major events of the 20th century. We all enjoyed looking at the pictures from a bygone era. Several books were published around this time as the world awaited in anticipation of Y2K, many fearing that computers would fail all over the globe, ending civilization as we now know it. It was then I realized how many years that Mom and people of her era had lived successfully without them.

When I started my teaching career at Iola Senior High School in Iola, Kansas, in 1973, I taught what was then called a mini-course in science fiction literature. Many futuristic books at that time predicted that the twenty-first century would be a time with many hours of leisure because of all the modern labor-saving devices. Many predictions were right on the mark, but the prediction of more leisure time was quite the opposite. I hardly ever hear of anyone now having too much leisure time on their hands. Before the advent of the two income family and the increased technology so that we can all be in constant contact with each other and the world, I can remember Mom having time to have a leisurely talk with our neighbor Corky while they both hung out the wash. We have also made so much so-called progress that we have to worry about whether or not it is legal to pray at public gatherings. So much has changed—for good and for bad.

Looking through the book, it occurred to me that since Mom was born in 1909, she had lived through all but a few years described in its pages. Geronimo had died the same year that Mom was born. She had lived through so much history I had only read about. She had lived in the era of the Model T, been through two visits of Haley's Comet, and all the wars from WWI to the Gulf War, Desert Storm. She was a young teenager when Babe Ruth made his home run records and when women won the right to vote.[10]

She was in high school during the flapper era. Her high school graduation picture sits on top of our entertainment center in an antique gold frame. Looking at it, she was always quick to tell me that some of her family members called her Bobby at that time since she was one of the first in town to bob or cut her long hair. The sepia toned picture doesn't show her rich lavender blouse that she had sewn herself that accented her deep blue eyes.

I could always remember that Charles Lindbergh flew the Atlantic in 1927 because Mom always told me that he was crossing the Atlantic in *The Spirit of St. Louis* on the day of her graduation tea at Parsons High School in Parsons, Kansas. I was always so proud that she and Dad had graduated from high school since it wasn't as common during that time period.

Mom and Dad had met in high school. She described

him as being tall with dark brown hair and huge blue eyes. She wrote his name down in her notebook the first day he came into class, and he started courting her soon after. Dad began his career on the M-K-T railroad in the shops, and Mom worked as a clerk at Cole's Department store after graduation. They dated for close to seven years, the last four during the Great Depression, before they finally got married. Back then, a man wouldn't think of asking a woman to marry him until he was financially stable, and he could adequately provide for her and a future family. When Dad finally did propose, he said something to the effect of, "Get your bills paid off, Cutes, and then we can get married."

Reviewing the century triggered other memories that Mom had told us about. In 1934, Bonnie and Clyde died in a police ambush in Louisiana. Her grandson Mark had memories of he and grandma playing Bonnie and Clyde in an old car parked in back of the house. Shirley Temple won her Oscar at the ripe old age of seven.[11] Eleven years later when I was born in 1945, Shirley was still in the hearts and minds of American mothers. Many wanted their daughters to be like Shirley. As a young child, Mom wanted me in fussy dresses with ribbons and bows, curly hair, ruffled socks, and black patent leather shoes. This was a natural lead into signing me up for tap and ballet lessons.

The book reviewing the twentieth century reminded me how much times have changed. Mom had celebrated her graduation as Lindbergh crossed the Atlantic. I graduated from high school in 1963, and the following November, at Parsons Junior College, I first heard the news of John F. Kennedy's assassination. Kennedy is well remembered for his great contributions to the space program and the race with Russia. I think it is true that most of us who were alive and old enough know exactly what they were doing when they heard the news about Kennedy that terrible day. I was practicing cheers in my mind in front of my locker, getting ready for a pep assembly for the Friday night football game. In the blur of faces and chaos of the hallways between classes, I heard "Kennedy has been shot." The pep assembly turned into a vigil of silence and prayer. Time stood still for a moment. It was a time of shock and loss of innocence for me and many young people in America with the subsequent assassination of Robert Kennedy and Martin Luther King. As Bob Dylan so aptly put it in his song, "The times they are a changing."

Through all the pages of all the books about the twentieth century, as well as all the pages of our lives, one thing remained constant. The rock we three kids had to hold onto was her unconditional love for all of us. The rock she held onto was her faith in Jesus as her savior. She reflected the kind of love that the Lord has for all who are willing to follow Him. This was her greatest gift to us as children and throughout our lives.

Letting Go

According to the professionals, no one dies directly from AD but from complications of the disease such as injury, infection, respiratory problems, dehydration, malnutrition, weakening from another chronic condition or a combination of the above. My mother had bouts with each of these from time to time. In spite of the fact that she was very physically healthy for someone her age, ninety, almost ninety-one, her body was simply wearing out from the ravages of age, as well as the insidious progression of AD.

About a year before she died in August of 2000, her appetite started to decrease dramatically. It is not uncommon for the elderly to experience a decrease in appetite with a subsequent decrease in activity. Mom's circumstances were just the opposite. Her appetite diminished at a time in her life when she felt a constant need to be on the move because of the AD. She didn't eat enough to fuel this increased activity, and so her weight continued to drop. I was told by the nursing home staff that many AD patients fail to interpret the physical signs of hunger, forget that they need to eat, or in some cases, the brain fails to tell them they are hungry.

It was then that I realized there was no way anyone can make another person eat, short of force feeding. No one, of course, would approve of this practice, but many staff members, myself, family members, as well as my husband Arley, did a great deal of coaxing during this time. Similar to a child, if she didn't want to eat, she would simply get up from the table and walk off. Over a year or so, we tried everything. Finally, one of the nurses said, "Is there any food or drink your mother really, really likes?" Offhandedly, I said, "Sure, beer!" She had always liked a beer on occasion, and she hadn't had any for a very long time. I expected to hear the nurse laugh; instead, she said, "We could get the doctor to order it." I thought she was kidding, but she said that beer was just as good to stimulate the appetite as wine. Of course, she would only get small amounts. That seemed reasonable to me.

When I got home in Miami, I went to a local liquor store to buy her a six pack of beer. All I saw in the beer case were twelve packs. Two six packs wasn't a bad idea. I could just take one six pack at a time to the nursing home, I reasoned. I definitely didn't want to lug in a twelve pack. The whole situation seemed a little bizarre to me anyway, but I was willing to try anything.

I said to the clerk, "Do you have two six packs? All I see in the beer case are twelve packs."

She looked at me like she couldn't believe what she was hearing. "Two six packs have the identical number of cans as one twelve pack, don't they?"

I knew my explanation would only complicate things, but I progressed on with the conversation. "My mom is in a nursing home, and I just wanted to take her one six pack at a time."

Then she looked at me like she was convinced that I had totally lost my mind. I was afraid that she might call the elder abuse hotline. After I explained the unusual situation, she laughed while putting the cans into two plastic six pack holders. The beer idea didn't work out either, but it was worth a try. Besides, I'm sure she enjoyed the one or two beers she had, probably as little as a half a can at a time.

In November of 1999, she became unresponsive due to dehydration and was taken to the hospital in Neosho. After a few days of hydrating her with an IV, she bounced back to normal in a matter of weeks. I even have a picture of her pushing another resident around in a wheel chair in March of 2000, around three months before she went into the hospital for the last time.

Arley's mom Ruth was eighty-two and a resident of Medicalodge also. For several years, every time the phone rang late at night, the sound would pierce my heart, wondering if this was "the call" for me or for Arley. The dreaded call finally came in June of 2000. Mom had once again become unresponsive. In my rush the forty minute drive to Neosho seemed longer than usual. In my heart I hoped that it would just be dehydration again like it was the November before, and that she would miraculously bounce back again. This was not to be.

I arrived about the same time the ambulance got there from Freeman Hospital in nearby Joplin, Missouri, and so I followed it back there. After I drove up to the emergency entrance, I searched for her Living Will and my Medical Power of Attorney papers. I kept them handy in my glove compartment. It was June 21, 2000, and as I glanced at the date on the POA, I noticed it was signed by both of us on exactly the same date six years before on June 21, 1994.

In June of 1994, she had been showing signs of memory loss for over a year. As the family looked back, it had probably been longer than that, but it became more obvious around that time. In the first stages of memory loss, I'm sure she did a great deal of covering up. She was always a person who wasn't afraid to laugh at her mistakes.

Around that time I started thinking about the future. She had already signed a Living Will on her own, and I was relieved that she was the one who brought up the subject of signing a Durable Power of Attorney and Medical Power of Attorney. She was a very intelligent and caring woman, and I was grateful that she had decided to make this most important decision on her own. I lived only an hour and ten minutes from her apartment in Parsons, and so I was the logical one to sign it. This made it so much easier for me and the rest of my family to know her wishes, and it was easier emotionally to do this very important business before she was in dire need of it.

In the waiting room of the attorney's office, she just wanted to make sure that signing a Living Will wasn't the same as allowing suicide. I assured her that signing it would just mean that when death was imminent, the medical people would do everything to save her life but would stop short of any heroic measures which would just prolong certain death. This was a very brave woman facing her worst fear AD, and yet caring for her soul and making future decisions that would make it easier for the family she loved.

That Wednesday night, she was unresponsive for the most part but would rise up from time to time in the emergency room, probably wondering what was going on. AD really does complicate hospital stays. Then she would drift back to sleep or perhaps semi-consciousness. For the next few days, she would be hydrated and somewhat nourished from an IV. She stayed unresponsive in this deep sleep for days, and the doctor at the hospital was convinced that she had little time to live. The medical staff at Freeman Hospital was so kind to us at this difficult time and even put her into a private room so that the family could gather round.

Traveling from some distance, my two brothers and their families came to be by her side for what we all thought would be the last time. Miraculously, Mom woke up that Saturday night and was able to communicate with family members for a few days. The following Monday afternoon she was moved back to Medicalodge. The IV's had made her stronger for a while, and I think that having her whole family there stimulated her to stay somewhat alert. Perhaps, this was just another awesome gift from God. Looking back, it was most likely a little bit of both.

Before she woke up, we were told that they could keep

her alive with IV's and a feeding tube almost indefinitely. We all knew what her wishes were and decided to leave her fate in the hands of the loving Lord. She would not have wanted to live that way without much quality of life. We were lucky our family had a chance to be together with her for a few more days. I was fortunate because I had just retired and was able to be with her as long as I wanted and needed.

One incident during this time really stands out in my mind. Her great-grandson Dustin was only nine years old at the time. I know it was a shock for him to see her that way. He expected to see her like she had been when they came to our farm several years before. The lush green of the trees and grass surrounded Spring River that rolled the length of our farm. The river settles itself around gently sloping hills thick with a great variety of trees, which include hardwoods like elm, maple, oak, as well as the yellow-green of the willow. Squeals of laughter echoed down Spring River as Mom and Dustin threw rocks into the water yelling, "One, two, three—go!" They let loose the stone on the last word, waiting to hear the splash and watching the ripples of water spread out into concentric circles. He expected to see her like the time I had to ask them to quiet down in bed because I had to go to work the next day. They both had on their animal house shoes. One had puppy feet and the other raccoon feet. In retrospect, I wish I had let them laugh all night if they wanted.

After a while, Dustin became a little restless, and I asked him if he would like to go for a walk outside. Like a typical nine-year-old, he walked by my side, ahead of me, behind me, on a rock ledge, exploring the world outside the nursing home. I knew that his parents had prepared him for the worse when he started talking about her going to heaven. I said that she had lived a very long time and that is just exactly what would happen eventually.

My brother Jon, his grandfather, is an electronic engineer, and so his son Mark always had computers around; consequently, Dustin had played with computers before he could even read. One day to his grandfather's surprise, at about the age of four, he clicked his way into a computer game by recognizing the icons. So, our conversation was a mixture of philosophy and spirituality, sprinkled with "computereze."

I tried to explain to Dustin about Alzheimer's disease by telling him that she was still a very smart woman but that she was confused at times because her memory didn't work like it used to. This, I explained, was why she didn't know people some of the time. He dropped his head and lowered his voice. With a sad face, he said, "Oh, I see, she lost her memory cards." I also explained that even though she didn't even know the most important people in her life sometimes that she never forgot the Lord. Something clicked in his young mind when he said, "Oh, she can still get through to Jesus.com!"

The doctor in the hospital had expected her to die there. After visiting her at Medicalodge, her primary care physician finally confirmed the fact that she had suffered from a subdural hematoma, which was the cause of her slurred speech and paralysis on one side of her body. The extent of the paralysis wasn't discovered until later because of her lack of movement due to dehydration and subsequent semi-consciousness. After arriving at Medicalodge, no one there expected her to live much longer. Instead, she lived another amazing five weeks. It was a long, hard wait for the entire family, but it did give us time to realize that she wouldn't have wanted to live that way without much quality of life.

As the weeks went by, I questioned why God would let her linger like that; yet, I still wasn't ready to let her go. She had already progressed slowly through the stages of AD over the past seven years, and now her dying was to be slow and excruciating also. I know it was selfish since she was the one suffering but I continued to question. How much can I stand?

As I look back, God in his wisdom had his own purpose

and special timing. It gave me time to think about my own mortality. It seems that when our parents and the generation before us dies off, we have to face that we are next. Although our basic personalities and approach to life were very different, I have always identified closely with her. She was five feet two inches tall while I'm around five feet four inches. I would look at her legs and notice that mine were the same shape but larger. I could see myself twenty or thirty years from now. Also, in those next five weeks, I learned to depend more and more on God, and there were blessings along the way.

Saying Goodbye

The two people who really kept me glued together during those long six weeks before my mother's death were my husband Arley and Evelyn, the nursing home administrator. I remembered back about our conflict when I tried to make Mom's room look like a picture in *Better Homes and Gardens*, totally ignoring the needs of the staff of the nursing home, as well as her next roommate. How trivial that was in comparison to what I was facing now. Evelyn reminded me that even in my time of grief, I needed to be aware that the nursing home staff was experiencing a loss also. Mom had been a resident there for over three and a half years, and the people who were close to her needed to say their goodbyes also. She explained that they had two losses—the resident, along with the family members they would no longer see on a regular basis after the death of their loved one.

The west wing was composed of the Alzheimer's unit while the east wing was primarily concerned with skilled nursing. I'm sure that several of the patients suffered dementia on the east wing also, but they were confined to their beds, wheelchairs, or slower movement because of physical ailments. Because of this, the fear of their wandering off undetected was a low priority. Most of the staff members on the east wing were familiar with Mom because of her escapades during the rehabilitation of her broken hip. Everyone was sad to see her so immobile.

Staff members also visited from the west or the Alzheimer's unit from time to time. They would come during their breaks, as well as before and after work. God had certainly led us to a loving environment. I remember three young girls especially—Bonnie, Brandy, and Carrie. Although Mom was only semi-conscious, they would hold her hand, talk to her, and offer to help give her baths or perform any other kind of service to help out. You must remember that they would be doing this on their own time. They didn't even work on that unit! My heart melted when Bonnie reminded me, "We love Margaret, too."

Two weeks before Mom's death, Judy, who single-handedly ran the nursing home beauty shop, asked if Margaret had any needs concerning her hair. She knew how Mom always liked to have her hair look the way it always had. Many people had commented over the years how beautiful her thick and luxurious silver hair was. It was important to me, too. In the stress of all the medical problems, it is probably hard for men to understand, but I wanted Mom's hair to look nice. To me the beauty of her hair was, at least, one thing that never changed. Also, all her life Mom would get depressed if her hair wasn't done. It seems that no matter how old a lady gets, she still wants to look as good as possible. Judy, the beautician, understood this and gave of her time to work at reduced rates to make elderly men and women hold onto some self-esteem. Because she gave of herself so joyfully, I know it was a calling from God.

In my mind I knew this would be the last time she was in the beauty shop. I also knew we were preparing her for burial. I didn't want someone at the funeral home who was unfamiliar with her hair to do it for the last time. I wanted it to look as normal as possible.

Judy's love and generosity reminded me of the story in the Bible about the woman at Bethany who anointed the head of Jesus with oil during His final days on earth in preparation for what was ahead. In Matthew Chapter 7: 1–13, we learn that while visiting Simon the Leper, a woman came to Him with a jar of perfume and poured it on his head. The disciples criticized her because this expensive perfume was worth about a year's wage. They thought that she should have sold the perfume and given the money to the poor. Jesus answers, "She has done a beautiful thing." Later He goes on to say, "When she poured this perfume on my body, she did it to prepare me for burial. I tell you the truth, wherever the gospel is preached throughout the world, what she has done will also be told, in memory of her." The acts of kindness performed by people like Judy, the hospital staff at Freeman, and the staff at Medicalodge are like the woman at Bethany who went far beyond what was expected of them because they have the love of Christ in their hearts.

So many relative strangers continued to give of themselves as the weeks dragged on. Mom's ninety-first birthday rolled around on July 15. Although she was becoming less and less aware of her surroundings, I decided to try to help her celebrate her birthday anyway. It was probably as much for myself as her, but I guess under the circumstances that was okay. I brought a large birthday sheet cake for both the east and west wings and left one for everyone else in the break room. It was as much to show my appreciation to the staff as anything.

Bonnie, Brandy, and Carrie, as well as several other staff members, came into her room to have cake and sang "Happy Birthday." It was sweet and very sad at the same time. I'm glad we celebrated anyway because I remember how much Mom had always liked birthdays. A few years before when she broke her hip, I remember zipping her down the hallway of Medicalodge in her wheelchair to dinner with birthday balloons flying behind.

I also remember a surprise party she had planned for me when I was only five years old. She had planned a circus theme, and the birthday cake was decorated like a carousel. It was hard to keep any illusions about life having two older brothers. They never could keep a secret. One brother exposed the Santa Claus myth almost before Mom had time to tell me the story about "The Night Before Christmas." So, it only figures that I knew about the surprise party long before it happened.

I could hardly sleep the night before picturing my friends bringing toys and candy in bright boxes. I'd make a wish and then blow out the pink candles on the cake that Mom had hidden on the top shelf of her closet. My brothers had already found it. Near the end of recess at school the following day, I was shocked to hear that not all my classmates had been invited to my surprise party. Hadn't Mom always said to be nice to everyone? Wasn't she the one who told me never to leave anyone out? This was an oversight soon to be corrected. I invited everyone in my homeroom plus anyone else I saw on my way home from school. Over fifty kids showed up. What a party! Boy, was Mom surprised.

Mom and Dad had hired a photographer for the party. So many kids tried to pack themselves into one area that he had to stand on a chair in the kitchen to take the picture of all the party goers overflowing into the dining room. It didn't occur to me until years later that she could actually have become irritated over the incident. She didn't. She just kept sending Dad out for more ice cream and cake. I thought of this as I took her cake around to everyone I could find in the facility.

During her last weeks at Medicalodge, the doctor had warned the family that her days were numbered and that she could pass on at any given time. Our family thought she would die in the hospital five weeks before, and then there was another scare about a week before she actually died. At this time it was no longer a question of "if" but "when." The following Monday, Dr. Hill came to visit and explained that her system was definitely shutting down. Although waiting for her to pass felt like the proverbial "insult on injury," I did learn to get strength from God. I began to understand more clearly how David felt when he spoke the following words in Psalms 18:1–2. "I love you, O Lord, my strength. The Lord is my rock, my fortress and my deliverer; my God is my rock, in whom I take refuge." As sad as I felt, I knew now that she was in God's hands and that God's timing was perfect. It was just my job to wait and be with her.

Most of my visits over the past three and a half years at Medicalodge had been during the day. Toward the end I even spent several nights at the facility because I didn't want her to be alone when she died. Even something good came out of this because I got to meet more people who had come to like her who worked at night when I was never around. One young CNA, Vickie, was especially kind, and she told me that her husband knew Margaret very well because he worked on the Alzheimer's unit on the west wing. Apparently, he found out that Mom liked Cheetos and had brought some to work for her on several occasions. I went to the west wing to thank him, and we all shared more Margaret stories.

On Wednesday, the day before her death, Martha, the director of nursing, together with Evelyn and her incredible sense of timing, temporarily moved Mom's roommate out that night so that Arley and I could be with her in private as long as we wanted. That afternoon I played the Mills Brothers tape and remembered how much fun we had that one spring day singing, *Up the Lazy River*, riding around Neosho and going for ice cream. Tears welled up in my eyes when the tape broke and the music stopped.

When death didn't come that day, I slept in the former roommate's bed, but Arley preferred sleeping in his truck in the parking lot instead of the recliner in her room. Being an outdoorsman, he liked the outside air better anyway, and it was definitely quieter. He had gone back to Miami after work, showered, brought clean clothes, and settled down for the night, being only about five minutes from his job.

Our whole family had been prepared so many times. Not knowing that she would actually die that Thursday evening (August 3, 2000), Arley went home to Miami, exhausted after work for a short nap before joining me later. As time passed, Mom's breathing became more and more labored. I looked down at her legs and saw signs of lack of circulation. The bluish-black had worked up to her ankles. In my mind I was saying, "God, I can't do this alone!" Just as I was leaving to inform the nearby nurses' station, I practically collided with Evelyn, the nursing home administrator, coming around the corner on her way to see us. This was God's timing again, I thought. Evelyn reminded me that the sense of hearing was the last to go. This was comforting to me because I wanted Mom to know that she wasn't alone.

As I look back, none of us had ever been alone. The Lord is always with us. For the next hour or so, I sat on the side of her bed with one arm on her shoulder and the other resting on her free hand. Evelyn and I talked, prayed, and waited. She had just asked me how Arley and I had met. Even in that sorrowful time, I must have had some joy in my voice. Maybe, somehow she knew I would be okay. When the time came, she looked at peace. I knew I would miss her more than I could miss anyone in my life. I also knew that she would see the face of the Lord and look at Him even more lovingly than she had looked at His picture as I saw her do so many times when I was growing up. After her spirit left her physical body, it struck me that she would now know who I was once again.

Remembering Margaret

In 1983, Mom left instructions for her funeral services in her safety deposit box. The outside of the envelop read: "To be opened after my death—funeral services. Do as I say or I'll come back and haunt you." Inside, she addressed it to "the best and most devoted children in the world." She must have known how hard it would be for us, and so she requested a very simple graveside service.

We planned a visitation at the funeral home from 9:30 to 10:30 with graveside services at 11:00. Of course, there were tears and sadness at the loss. In addition, there were many wonderful memories. We had all gathered in somewhat of a circle, each talking in small groups. As time went on, we merged together and quite spontaneously started telling Margaret stories.

Mayellen was a close relative and next door neighbor all the time we were growing up in that old house on Kennedy Street in Parsons. It had been a duplex, but the wall was knocked down to form one very large living room instead of two separate ones. This meant that we had duplicate entrances on both ends of the house. This also meant that we had two front porches with a concrete slab in between with a set of steps going up to each one.

On several different occasions, when a salesman would ring the doorbell on the west side, Mom would answer the door bell with Mayellen sitting on the living room couch.

Mom would say, "I don't want anything right now, but you might ask the lady next door." The salesman would go down one set of stairs and up the other to be greeted by Mom at the other door and Mayellen sitting on the other couch. Mom would then say, "We don't want any either."

Everyone remembered the day when the daughter of one of the prominent local doctors came to our house to visit. Halfway into lunch, our boxer Duke left the comfort of his easy chair to chase the neighbor's cat off the front porch, taking a short cut through our living room window. Fortunately, Dad was downtown paying bills. He had somewhat of a temper at times, especially on bill paying day. Mom hurried to phone the glass company as one of my brothers yelled, "Please, don't get rid of Duke. I'll pay for the window out of my allowance. I'll get a paper route after school." Dad had said that if Duke broke anything else in the house that he would have to go.

About that time the doctor's daughter spotted Dad coming up the walk. Always a quick thinker in a crisis, Mom grabbed the grocery list and sent him to the store. When he returned home an hour later, she sent him to the pharmacy. She made the glass man park in front of the neighbor's house when he came and then insisted he duck down out of view each time my dad came home. By the time the window was replaced, she had run my dad all over town. The glass man finally left exhausted from the rushing, prodding, and hiding just minutes before Dad came home ragged from his last errand with the weekly dry cleaning in hand. I always laughed at the *I Love Lucy* TV shows, but I could also relate to the predicaments she got into like my mother did.

The doctor and his wife pulled up behind Dad in their shiny new car; they had come to pick up their daughter. When Mom requested that my friend come back soon, she squealed, "I sure will. Nothing exciting ever happens at our house."

Stories continued to fill the empty spaces in our hearts

with laughter. Nothing planned would have been a more fitting tribute to my mother than to remember her in love and laughter.

 We all got into our cars and made the long procession through Parsons to the graveside services on the other side of town. After the services, the great-grandchildren gathered by the casket while Dustin, with Erik and Kevin at his side, put one rose on top with a red ribbon. The golden letters read, "My Bestest Buddy." Although a simple service, it brought out two very important aspects of her life—her legacy of laughter and her great love for children.

A New Beginning

I had promised the Lord several years before that if He would help me get through my mother's decline and death that I would start going to church as soon as my job of taking care of her needs was over. It seemed reasonable at that time, but I was wrong on several different counts. For one thing, I'm not sure it's such a good idea to bargain with the Lord. I know now that I should turn to Him for guidance and not play *Let's Make a Deal*. Another important thing I learned is that I would have been so much better off over those seven years had I attended all along. My priorities had been wrong. It was like I had run the race of dealing with my mother's AD, decline, and death and then waited until it was over to reflect on how I should have run it. By joining a church, I would have had the support of a Christian community and a church home. At the very least, I had made the right decision to start going to church now.

I had been away from church for so long that I wasn't even sure what denomination I wanted to attend. I wanted to find a church that my husband and I would both feel comfortable in. Arley's father had been a Pentecostal minister while I had attended the First Christian Church in Parsons, Kansas, as well as the Episcopal Church. We were to move to our lake lot in Grove, Oklahoma, as soon as the farm was sold. We were getting older and wanted to scale down. It made sense to look for a church there. Elk River Baptist Church was close to where we planned to move, and so I decided to go there the following Sunday after Mom's funeral on the previous Monday.

In my mind a promise was a promise, especially to the Lord. I think He would have understood if I had waited a week to catch my breath, especially after my very long absence. I didn't know anyone who attended that church, and my emotions were still very raw with grief when I walked in the door. I thought the church services started at 10:00, but Sunday school started at 10:00, and church started at 11:00. Since I was already there, I was naturally invited to Sunday school. I went into the women's class. When my first husband died, I hadn't attended church for a while, but when I did on several different occasions, I would become very emotional. After my mother's passing, the same thing still held true. When a lady in the class mentioned heaven, I started to cry. It was then I had to explain that my mother had just passed away. They were very sweet and said a prayer for my mom and me.

I kept myself together in church, and then walking out the door, I saw a Grove teacher I had known from when I had lived there before. She asked me if I was still teaching to which I replied, "I retired last May." Carol was probably one of the sweetest and most tender hearted people I knew and wouldn't hurt a soul for a million dollars. Not knowing, she asked the natural question, "How are you enjoying your retirement so far?" My mind flashed back to all I had gone through that summer with Mom's illness and death, and I started crying again. I felt like such an idiot. After I got my composure, I explained my outburst and apologized for making her feel uncomfortable.

Although this had been a rather rocky and embarrassing start, it turned out to be the perfect choice for me. I didn't know much about the Baptist faith, but I liked the people because they were so loving and positive, and I really felt the presence of God in that church. I'm not saying that everyone should join the Baptist church. This was just a good choice for me at the time. Most of all, the pastor, Dan Dareing, seemed so alive with his love for Christ in a real way.

I had never regularly attended a church that had an invitation at the end of the service. Baptist churches, as well as several other Protestant churches, provide an opportunity at the end of the worship service for people to make public their commitment to Jesus. It is based on Matthew 10:32. Jesus said, "Whosoever acknowledges me before men, I will also acknowledge him before my Father in heaven. But whosoever disowns me before men, I will disown him before my Father in heaven."

I sat through one invitation after another for the next several weeks, each time feeling a slight tug to go forward. Then one Sunday morning the most amazing thing happened. At the beginning of the invitation, Brother Dan said that if anyone had a burden to lay on the altar to come forward. I found out later that a young man named Scott had left in an agitated state, went to his car to leave, and saw a beer can in his back seat. At that moment he decided to come back into the church and give his concerns to God. All I saw was this young man walking down the aisle placing an empty can of beer on the altar. I didn't know anything about his circumstances, but I thought that if he could do that in public, surely I could go forward. At that split second, I felt like something grabbed the collar of my blouse and pulled me forward to the front. Before I knew it, I was repeating the *Sinners Prayer*.

"Jesus, I am a sinner and I ask forgiveness of my sin according to Your loving sacrifice on the cross and Your powerful resurrection. I humbly ask You to save me now from the penalty of sin, hell, death, and the grave. I invite You to come into my heart and be the Lord of my life. I believe in my heart that You died for my sins and God has raised you from the dead. I am no longer ashamed of You and I thank You for eternal life. From this moment forward,

I will serve You. Please take complete control of my life for Thou art my God and my Savior. Thank You for saving me right now in Jesus Name. Amen."

After going forward at church, a few more Sundays passed. In Oklahoma, September is still a very warm month. The church ceiling is extremely high with huge brass and glass lights spaced out all over its wide expanse. Between these lights are ceiling fans to force the air to circulate evenly. On each of the ceiling fans is a cluster of lights with a short chain to switch the fans off and on. The ceiling is much too high to use these short chains, and so they are all controlled by a main switch on the north side of the sanctuary. When the fans reach a certain speed, the chains hit the glass on the light globes at unpredictable intervals. The hitting of the chains on the glass globes sounds like the clear tinkling of crystal bells. I know it was just my imagination, but I liked to think that the sound was my mother saying "hello." I couldn't help but smile every time it happened. A few Sundays later, as Brother Dan started speaking of heaven, several bell sounds took their turns giving off their crystal clear clinks. Amused at the coincidence, he stopped for a moment and said something to the effect that he was glad to have the tinkling of the bell sounds punctuate his message.

Again according to Baptist doctrine, the first act of obedience is to be baptized into the faith. On September 24, I decided it was time. I was a little nervous sitting in the pew with my husband Arley that Sunday night waiting to be immersed in the water. About that time the bell sounds from the fan lights started to tinkle in various places all over the church. Gary, the music director, unobtrusively walked to the main switch to try to find a speed that would quiet the ringing. He tried several times before they were finally silenced. I laughed to myself and thought it was just Mom's way of showing her approval. It was always hard to quiet her down when she was excited. It was almost like she was applauding. The sound was very reassuring, and it made me feel even more secure in my decision. Several Sundays later, Brother Dan gave a sermon in which he emphasized Hebrews 12:1. "Therefore, since we are surrounded by such a great cloud of witnesses, let us throw off everything that hinders and the sin that so easily entangles, and let us run with perseverance the race marked out for us."

When I first walked into that church, I was forced to cope with the finality of my mother's life on earth. Several Sundays after my baptism and the wild tinkling of the bells, I listened in amazement as I heard Brother Dan say that he believed that all the faithful who had gone before us, including Moses and David, were cheering us on. My mother had given me physical life fifty-five years before, and now I believe that she was cheering me on to the beginning of my new spiritual life with the Lord as my guide, a commitment she had made so many years before.

Set Me Adrift

This book was meant to explore only one person's unique experience in dealing with the ravages of Alzheimer's disease.

Everyone with Alzheimer's is different. The saying, "When you've seen one person with Alzheimer's, you've seen ONE person with Alzheimer's" couldn't be more true. However, most caregivers will agree that during the course of the disease, there are similarities and universal challenges that almost all will eventually face.[12]

Our family was fortunate, in a way, because my mother was easier to deal with than some who are afflicted. Although she definitely had her moments of agitation, she didn't rage or lash out for the most part. Because she was small, she was easier to redirect. Her unusual physical well-being for her age caused a few problems but spared us from the heartache of seeing her in a wheelchair or confined to bed over a long period of time. In many ways she was more fortunate than some stricken with AD, but naturally watching her mental and physical deterioration was still heart wrenching, to say the least.

It is always hard to see a family member lose a grasp of who they are. The opposite is also true. I have talked to people whose family member or loved one had the mental capacity to fully comprehend a future with little or no hope for survival. I don't know which is worse. Both are difficult to endure. Pain is pain, no matter what the source.

As we are all very aware, life on earth is full of struggles of all kinds. Dealing with the difficulties we face in life can make us bitter, or it can bring us closer to God. Through my struggle, I started to see that God had a plan for my life, even if it wasn't always clear to me what it was. My teaching experience and my counseling degree brought me a great deal of understanding about the world, but spirituality was the key to finding real meaning in life and peace in my heart.

One of the most positive aspects of this experience occurred whenever I could help someone else who had a friend or family member dealing with AD or some other related disorder. Through this book, I wanted to reach people and give them hope that something, which at first may seem to be devastating, can help you learn life's lessons, make you stronger, and bring you closer to God. I hope this book has brought you a measure of comfort if you are going through a very trying time.

The seven years I dealt with my mother's AD was a spiritual journey. During one of our long lunches and literary discussions, my writer friend Joan Isom reminded me that writing a book is also a journey. I will always miss my mother with all my heart. However, writing this book has helped put my life and my mother's life into perspective for me. Through putting my feelings and experiences into writing, I soon came to the conclusion that there was no one else quite like my mother. The way she made us laugh and the way she loved all her children unconditionally was just a normal accepted part of our lives. Now, I realize that she was a special gift from God that we were all so blessed to enjoy. Shame flushed my face when it occurred to me that I had never thanked God for her. My life would have been so different had she been different. Putting together the pieces of the puzzle of my life with her has provided me closure and healing.

Several months have passed since my mother's death, and slowly calmness and joy have come back into my heart. I compare those seven years of struggle with my mother's AD to having someone step on my foot for a very long time. When the foot was finally removed, it felt so good. All I could think of for a while was grief but also a sense of relief that my mother no longer had to suffer on this earth. My mind was so full of the past and present that I had little time to focus on the future.

Recently, Rhonda, one of the members of our church, gave an inspirational talk and sang a beautiful song about Jesus helping us through the storms of our lives. Unknown to her until a phone call the night before, Brother Dan planned to talk about Jesus calming the waters on that very same Sunday.

During his sermon, Brother Dan made the comment that all of us have either just passed through one of life's storms, are currently experiencing one, or one may be looming on the horizon. With the history of dementia in our family, I was forced to come to grips with the fact that the next storm could be mine.

A few weeks before my mother died, I had a dream about my being diagnosed with AD. When the doctor broke the news to me, I said, "I would rather put a gun to my head right now." Upon awakening, I started to think with my rational mind. Being a Christian means letting God use me in any way He sees fit. In a more recent sermon, Brother Dan commented that, "God doesn't deliver us from the storm; He delivers us in the storm." In other words, being a Christian doesn't keep up from having problems in life, but it does give us a savior and friend to lean on when times get tough.

Along with everyone else, I desperately hope for a cure for AD in my lifetime. But if it doesn't come in time for me, I must accept that also. I reasoned that if it is God's will that I go down the same road as my mother, I hope that I will be an inspiration to someone else, as she has been to me. The most important thing she taught me is that no matter what happens in life, Jesus will always have His hand in mine.

Set Me Adrift in the Sea of Faith

Set me adrift in the sea of
of faith, O Lord.
Give me the strength to endure
unspeakable loss and pain.
Replace my fear of the unknown
with hopeful expectation.
Help me let go of doubt, pride,
and my overwhelming need to control.
Ease me to that peaceful shore
and wrap me in a blanket of your love.
I long to hear you say,
"Be still, my child.
I am with you always."

Judith Ames David

I tell you the truth, unless you change and become like children you will never enter the kingdom of heaven.

Matthew 18:3

Endnotes

1. *The Dance.* Performed by Garth Brooks. Written by Tony Arata. Copyright 1989, Morganactive Songs, Inc./EMI. April Music Inc. (c/o Morgan Music Group, Inc.) ASCAP. Warner Bros. Publications (Print Agent).
2. Tammie J. Crispino, ed. *The Centennial Story of Parsons, Kansas.* (Parsons, Kansas: The Sun Graphics, Inc., 1971.
3. *The Dance.*)
4. Phyllis Young, "Shells," Newsletter. Used by permission of the Alzheimer's Association (Tulsa, Oklahoma Chapter).
5. Elisabeth Kubler-Ross, *On Death and Dying* (New York: Macmillan Publishing Co., 1969).
6. Maureen Reagan, Interview with Charlie Gibson and Diane Sawyer, *Good Morning, America*, ABC, New York.
7. Maureen Reagan interview.
8. Madeleine L'Engle, *The Crosswicks Journal: Book Two, The Summer of the Great-grandmother* (San Francisco: HarperCollins, 1974), p 51.
9. Anne Graham Lotz, *The Vision of His Glory: Finding Hope Through the Revelation of Jesus Christ*, Videotape and Workbook (Nashville, Tennessee: LifeWay Press, 1999).
10. Charles Phillips, Neil Grant, *et al.*, *The 20th Century Year by Year: The People and Events That Shaped the Last Hundred Years* (London: Marshall Publishing, 1999).
11. Phillips, Grant, *et, al.*
12. "When Someone You Know Has Alzheimer's." PRWeb (Press Release News Wire), Jupiter, Florida, 2004. Retrieved Oct. 17, 2006 from http://www.prweb.com/Releases/2004.

Bibliography

Crispino, Tammie J., ed. *The Centennial Story of Parsons, Kansas.* Parsons, Kansas: The Sun Graphics, Inc., 1971.

The Dance. Performed by Garth Brooks. Written by Tony Arata. Copyright 1989, Morganactive Songs, Inc./EMI. April Music Inc. (c/o Morgan Music Group, Inc.). ASCAP. Warner Bros. Publications (Print Agent).

Kubler-Ross, Elisabeth. *On Death and Dying.* New York: Macmillan Publishing Co., 1969.

L'Engle, Madeleine. *The Crosswicks Journal: Book Two. The Summer of the Great-grandmother.* San Francisco: HarperCollins, 1974.

Lotz, Anne Graham. *The Vision of His Glory: Finding Hope Through the Revelation of Jesus Christ.* Video and Workbook. Nashville, Tennessee: LifeWay Press, 1999.

Maier, Mary Anne and Joan Shaddox Isom, eds. *The Leap Years: Women Reflect on Change, Loss, and Love.* Boston: Beacon Press, 1999.

Phillips, Charles, Neil Grant, et. al. *The 20th Century Year by Year: The People and Events That Shaped the Last Hundred Years.* London: Marshall Publishing, 1999.

Reagan, Maureen. Interview with Charlie Gibson and Diane Sawyer. *Good Morning America.* ABC News. New York.

"When Someone You Know Has Alzheimer's." PRWeb (Press Release News Wire), Jupiter, Florida, 2004. Retrived Oct. 17, 2006 from http://www.prweb.com Releases/2004.

Young, Phyllis. *Shells.* Newsletter. Used by permission of Alzheimer's Association. (Tulsa, Oklahoma Chapter).